Lilo —
May God b
you —   Marlene

LEARNING TO
LIVE AGAIN IN A
NEW WORLD

LEARNING TO LIVE AGAIN IN A NEW WORLD

A Journey from Loss to New Life

Marlene Anderson, M.A.

ELM HILL

A Division of
HarperCollins Christian Publishing

www.elmhillbooks.com

Learning to Live Again in a New World

A Journey from Loss to New Life

Published in Nashville, Tennessee, by Elm Hill, an imprint of Thomas Nelson. Elm Hill and Thomas Nelson are registered trademarks of HarperCollins Christian Publishing, Inc.

Author Contact:
409 Umatilla Pl.
La Conner, WA 98257
360-466-3054 (phone number)
focuswithmarlene@gmail.com
www.focuswithmarlene.com

Elm Hill titles may be purchased in bulk for educational, business, fund-raising, or sales promotional use. For information, please e-mail SpecialMarkets@ ThomasNelson.com.

Library of Congress Cataloging-in-Publication Data

Library of Congress Control Number: 2019913424

ISBN 978-1-400329366 (Paperback)
ISBN 978-1-400329373 (Hardbound)
ISBN 978-1-400329380 (eBook)

" ... but they who wait upon the Lord shall renew their strength, they shall mount up with wings like eagles, they shall run and not be weary, they shall walk and not faint."

ISAIAH 40:31

CONTENTS

PART IV: A NEW BEGINNING

DEDICATION

This book is dedicated to LeRoy, my husband, confidant and best friend, and to all those who struggle to create a new life after a major loss and reach out to find comfort and hope for their future.

ACKNOWLEDGEMENTS

I want to thank everyone – friends and family – who helped me during my journey through grief and loss. We all loved Le Roy and he is missed by many.

And a special thank you to Ron Jones for the use of his studio, SkyMuse, in recording the audio portion of this book. Ron, you and Laree are very special to me.

And another thanks to Kyle Baker and Steven McAnulty, my audio engineers who persevered as I did the audio retakes during recording. You are great.

PREFACE

G rieving was some of the hardest work I have ever done. When my husband died after forty-two happy years of marriage, I looked for resources to help me through the process. The books available at the time were either too clinical or too singular in focus, such as biographies and memoirs. There were books that contained comprehensive information on the subject of grief and loss, but they required more energy than I had to chart a course in application. Support groups offered little in the way of strategies to help me move forward.

Using the knowledge and training I had as a psychology teacher and therapist, I created my own roadmap to letting go, assessing who I was after my loss and moving from one reality to another. I didn't just want to heal—I wanted to find a way to live again. Processing a loss is more than just recovery; it is redefining who you are in order to create a new beginning.

As I worked with grief and loss groups in my church, I found that individuals attending also wanted more information. While sharing stories with each other was helpful, they wanted tools and resources they could apply to their own individual walks of life.

There is no linear path through grief, and everyone's experience will be different, relevant to each specific situation. Our personalities, past experiences, gender, and the individual importance of our losses will determine our journeys. My expression of grief may not be your expression, but within its context we find both the personal and universal. There is a similarity in the process that can be applied to each unique situation.

Healing from losses requires more than just talking about our pain; it involves working through the twists and turns of conflicting emotions and confronting questions that often have no satisfactory answers. It is reassembling the pieces of life that have been shattered by assumptions and expectations.

There is a spiritual as well as emotional, physical, and psychological side to grieving. Our beliefs will be challenged. Is there an afterlife? Is there a God or Supreme Being? Both believers and unbelievers will be challenged because losses reveal our immortality and vulnerability. They strip away carefully constructed facades and confront us with the question, "Who am I?"

While this book is the culmination of my journey from loss to constructing new meaning for my life, it also offers information, questions, and exercises in the personal worksheets. The vignettes are snapshots from my journal depicting the painful thoughts and emotions associated with my grief walk. Together they can provide a source of both validation and a method to personalize another's journey.

The book is divided into four sections. "Part I: An Unwanted Journey" addresses those early days, weeks, and months when we feel the acute pain from our loss. "Part II: Letting Go: Closing the Door" identifies what is required to move forward. "Part III: From One Reality to Another: Redefining Yourself" asks the question, "Who am I now?" The final section, "Part IV: A New Beginning," suggests the many ways we can start a new chapter in our life stories. The "Appendixes" give more in-depth information on the grief and loss process, support systems, and dealing with difficult grief emotions.

Within our grief work, we begin to heal and recover. We will struggle with hanging on to what we had before we can let go. Eventually, we are able to close one chapter of life so another can begin. Healing does not mean we forget or no longer remember; it neither diminishes nor eliminates our losses. But it does mean we make conscious choices to move forward and our lives are no longer dominated by grief. We not only heal but find a new song and dance for our lives as well.

Marlene Anderson, M.A.

Part I
An Unwanted Journey

CHAPTER 1

THIS CAN'T BE HAPPENING

"Draw near to God and he will draw near to you."

JAMES 4:8

This can't be happening. There was so little warning. He had been so healthy. There was no time to prepare. I'm numb. What do I do now?

I no longer cry. I have already shed so many tears. All that remains is emptiness and the knowledge that I have just begun a very long journey. It's not one I thought I would be making at this time in my life. Although friends surround me, I realize I am the only one who can walk this road.

My husband of forty-two years has succumbed to the aggressive brain tumor. We had been so happy together over the years. I never imagined, even in my wildest dreams, he would be taken just as we had left the busy world of teaching and were settled into a semi-retirement lifestyle. How do I take the next step without him? Our lives had been intertwined in so many ways; who am I without him?

The pain becomes acute as the numbness recedes. If I am going to heal, I can't push the pain away or deny its existence. I can't run away. But everything inside me is screaming, *No! I don't want to let go. I don't want to have to do this.*

As reality sinks to a new level, I realize that my life has been changed forever. How do I start over? Do I stay in this beautiful home we just built, our dream house, or will I be required to sell it and move? We used to assess options and determine what to do together. Now, even with the caring advice of friends and family, I am responsible for everything. What if I make bad choices and lose everything?

I can only stay in the house for short periods of time before I flee to find solace outdoors. Somehow, it is easier to feel that things will be okay when I can smell the pungent earth on the trails in the woods or deeply breathe in the clean fresh air of early morning. Flowers are blooming on my deck, but they have lost their ability to stir my heart. Even their brilliance and beauty is lost and dulled by shock and pain.

Lord, you've said if we draw near to you, you will draw near to us. I am drawing near to you. Grant me strength and courage. Give me wisdom and enduring faith. Help me through these days.

Reflection and Personal Application

Our first reaction to any kind of trauma, crisis, or unexpected major loss is usually shock, disbelief, and anger. The world as we knew it has just ended. A part of us rebels and screams, "No!" Denial comes storming into our consciousness as we try to wrap our brain around what has happened.

The loss that set my world reeling came from the unexpected death of my husband. Yours might be the result of an unexpected divorce, the death of a child, or a debilitating injury or illness. You may feel as I did—that your life has just ended.

Our thoughts can go from *I can't believe this is happening to he was too young to die.* Or you might be thinking, *how he could do this to me and the kids. How will we survive? What will I do now?* Whatever the loss, there will be thoughts and feelings that create anxiety about the future and our ability to cope, survive, and start again. We feel alone and vulnerable.

A major loss is a journey into the wilderness. You have never been here before. You search desperately for information from your past to cling to and somehow apply to this situation. There have been anxiety-producing unknowns and realities in the past that have taken you through hills and valleys. But this does not fit with previous losses. This is so much more.

As shock wears off and the intensity and depth of our loss becomes more acute, we will find ourselves fatigued, barely able to meet the basic needs of the day. Be kind to yourself. You have suffered an injury.

Consider the following during this early time period:

1. Give yourself permission to move slowly. In those early days and weeks, shock provides a cushion that allows us to function. We may feel like a zombie or robot—going through the motions of day-to-day living without feeling. Everything may seem superficial, even when we are in the company of friends. As I wrote in my book, *A Love So Great, A Grief So Deep*, "You can laugh, enjoy their company, and yet, it is as though you were fractured—split—and another you is doing these things. The real you cannot feel".

2. Take time to rest and do less. Energy is depleted and everyday routines and jobs are often a struggle. It is difficult to focus and think. Even the simplest chores can be exhausting.

3. Accept help from others who offer their love and assistance. Be kind to yourself and allow others to be kind to you. You have been emotionally wounded. There are bandages for physical wounds. The bandage for an emotional wound is love and compassion. Others may not know the depth of your wound, but they care and want to help.

4. Remain in the present. Focus on what is necessary and expedient. As shock wears off, it is replaced with a more acute pain. Resist the temptation to think about what you might have done, what you didn't do, or what you did do. There will be time later to wrestle with questions. For now, simply allow yourself to "be."

5. Make a decision to deal with old or on-going family disputes when life has become more stabilized. Traumatic events can put a strain on any family relationship. Past disagreements, quarrels, and confrontations often surface, increasing levels of distress. Long-standing family feuds and differences can make this period of time more difficult.

CHAPTER 2

ALICE'S SURREAL WORLD

"God, you pulled me out of the grave, gave me another chance
at life when I was down-and-out."

PSALM 30:3 *THE MESSAGE*

I feel like I've fallen into an *Alice in Wonderland* hole where the rabbit
with his ticking watch runs in and out repeating, "It's late, it's late," and
you know it is your own ticking clock. Has life as I knew it, with easy conversation, circles of friends and a predictable future gone forever? Is this
the end of everything I treasured? Has the reality I knew gone for good?

Alice's size shrinks and expands as does mine. When I psyche myself
up, ready to take on this new world, I grow large, confident, hopeful,
energized, and able to do anything. When I drink the shrinking potion
that matches the changes I need to make that will enable me to enter
new doors, I am diminished in size and hear the echoes of my own voice
repeat, "Your life of constancy and reliability is over. There will never be
happy days again." And I fall further into the hole of hopelessness where
obstacles of creating a new beginning loom larger than monster shadows
on the wall.

It is here I meet the Cheshire cat who smiles with understanding of
my plight but quickly disappears as I move toward new relationships and

possibilities leaving only the illusion of a new and happy future. It is part of the surreal world I have fallen into. Life as I had known it, colored with love and companionship, is gone. Death has thrown me into a new existence where everything has changed and glimpses of a promising tomorrow fade as quickly as the Cheshire cat, who leaves behind a mocking grin.

Like Alice, I find myself scurrying about, trying to find a way out of this rabbit's hole of illusion and unreality. There must be a way to have normalcy again. Arriving at the Mad Hatter's tea party, I recognize myself in the frantic activities; hurrying here, there, and everywhere, trying desperately to find a slice of familiarity and predictability that will provide nourishment to my soul.

But as I lift my cup to drink, I find the cup broken and unable to hold the tea. The party of life has passed me by. And like Alice, I desperately try to return to the world I knew before death toppled me, a world where I was secure within a loving relationship. I find myself crying, "Wake up, wake up! Wake up from this strange land. Wake up to find your loved one with you once more. Wake up to the world you once knew."

I pray, "God, please take me out of this Alice in Wonderland world. Pull me out of this morass of grief and despair. I want to experience happiness again."

Reflection and Personal Application

In the blink of an eye, our world can be turned upside down and inside out, leaving us spinning like a top—stunned, bewildered, and in shock. The world as you had known it no longer exists. The sun shines brightly, traffic speeds past, and children laugh and squeal with delight. But you are numb to the sights and sounds around you. You move within the familiar sphere of your life, but you are no longer a participant, only an observer, on the outside looking in. You have fallen into a new existence where everything seems strange and unreal. While once you felt strong and confident, you now feel bewildered, inadequate and vulnerable.

Losses can be messy, confusing, and rarely straightforward. Like Alice, you may feel as though you have fallen into a new world of distorted fragments of what used to be. As you grieve, your life takes on a new dimension; besides working through the pain you are trying to make sense of what happened and somehow come to terms with it.

Processing any major loss is a progression that gradually moves us from one place in time to another. This Alice in Wonderland world you have fallen into has roads leading everywhere with no designated direction or destination. We are required to work through the confusion and disorder in order to gain a new clarity, purpose and perspective of our life and ourselves.

Minor losses are absorbed without a lot of thought or attention. We feel bad, make corrections, and then move on. The more intertwined and linked together with what we have lost, the more we may experience feelings of detachment and disconnection; the deeper the emotional attachment, the greater the adjustment.

On this journey through uncharted territory, you may experience visits from your loved ones. There were a number of times early in my grief walk when I felt the presence of my husband and "heard" him speak to me in my mind. My husband and I shared a close and compatible relationship. These events occurred when I least expected them, and I was surprised at how comforting they were. I shared these experiences in my first book, *A Love So Great, A Grief So Deep*, and mention them again because others I have spoken with have encountered similar incidents. They are not unusual.

You may also experience Déjà vu moments. I remember walking into the airport several months after the death of my husband to pick up my adult kids and was struck with an incredible sense that my husband would be walking down the tarmac to meet me. It was such a vivid and unexpected episode that I could hardly move or contain my intense grief. Anything connected in some significant way with our past can trigger an emotional response to the pain of today. Remember, these are only fleeting moments and will pass.

Some suggestions to consider:

1. It takes time and energy to heal. Give yourself permission to go slowly. Our culture gives us little time to mourn before we are required to return to work. Chores and responsibilities of family life demand attention. In our haste to remove ourselves from the grip of pain, we often push grief away. Grief that is denied the opportunity and time needed to be expressed and mourned will go underground and become corrosive to our bodies and spirits. At some point, it demands our attention.

2. Find a way to release overwhelming emotions. Allow the tears to fall. Talk with loved ones. Journaling is an excellent way to release all those intense, confusing, and muddled feelings. Writing helps give shape and form to our thoughts, bringing clarity and perspective. Taking it out of our minds and putting it down on paper helps to make them more manageable. Don't worry about how you write or what you put down. Just write what you are feeling and thinking in the moment. Journaling is for your eyes only, unless you wish to share.

3. Expect unanticipated moments. A song, a particular smell, a sound, a movie, and other situations may suddenly and unexpectedly trigger our loss with such intensity and pain that it takes our breath away. Allow the tears to fall. It is part of the process.

4. Welcome unforeseen "visits" from your loved one. It might be a fleeting "vision". It might be a vivid and startling dream. Most of these visits occur in the early days and months. Most people who have experienced such events have found them comforting and consoling. There is much we do not understand or comprehend about the spiritual realm. Such situations are real, even if we can't totally describe or explain them.

CHAPTER 3

A PSALM OF TEARS

"I cry out in the night before thee.
Let my prayer come before thee; incline thy ear to my cry."

PSALM 88:1–2

"I'm standing my ground, God, shouting for help, at my prayers
every morning, on my knees each daybreak. For as long as I
remember I've been hurting, I've taken the worst you can hand
out and I've had it... I'm bleeding, black and blue."

PSALM 88:13–16 *THE MESSAGE*

It is a psalm of tears, crying out for God's help. It is a psalm I highlighted in my Bible and wrote beside it my own pleas to God when my
loved one was dying. It was Holy Week, and I felt as though I was falling
into a dark abyss, a bottomless pit where there is no hope, only continual
sorrow. There were no promises for tomorrow. My world was disintegrat-
ing, and I felt as though God had abandoned me.

Psalm 88 continues to speak to me as I cry out in my grief. Where
are you God? When will the pain of loss subside? When will I wake up
from this nightmare and see new avenues of life? I feel as though I've
been punched black and blue. Since my husband's death, the layers of

loss continue to reveal themselves every morning. My heart aches, and it seems at times as if I am dying too.

As I reflect this morning on all that has happened, I wonder if in our walks with God we are not only learning how to live but also how to die. After all, aren't we required to die in many ways, not just physically, but also to destructive behaviors, thoughts, and attitudes that will eventually destroy us if we hang on to them? We die emotionally and at times spiritually. And we look for a model of resurrection, rebirth, and renewal not only for after death but here on earth as well. However, when I am in the throes of pain, I don't want to think of the grand scheme of things. I only want to be free of the pain.

I turn the page in my Bible and receive answers to my questioning mind through the words of a new Psalm. With tenderness, the Psalmist declares how much God cares for us, and I find my heart responding to that love.

"Your love, God, is my song and I'll sing it! I'm forever telling
everyone how faithful you are. I'll never quit
telling the story of your love ..."

PSALM 89:1–2 *The Message*

Reflection and Personal Application

Every morning during those early months of grief, I spent time on my deck. I came with my bible and journal. It was summer and the hummingbirds and potted plants would quiet my spirit. Sometimes, it would be evening or afternoons before I could find those quiet moments to spend with God and my pain. As I journaled, I experienced comfort and peace but also times of deep distress while searching for answers to questions that I had difficulty forming. Each day new thoughts would surface that directed my writing.

Grieving is an emotional and spiritual journey and at times we might feel as though we are dying. We take in details but are indifferent to what is happening around us. Particular times of day can trigger more intense pain or sorrow.

We experience a whole range of emotions in grief: shock, disbelief, despair, sadness, sorrow, anxiety, fear, anger, guilt, shame, and relief to name a few. At first, shock, disbelief, and denial leave us feeling numb, empty, devoid of feelings. As shock wears off, pain sets in, often accompanied by a pervasive and encompassing depression. We might feel relief that a loved one has died after a long struggle with illness and then feel guilt and shame for feeling that way. Conflicting emotions of relief and guilt also happens when a tragic accident allows us to live while a loved one dies.

As we travel through our grief journeys, we might experience hope and then hopelessness, pleasure and moments of contentment and then despair. Intensity and duration of emotions will vary from time to time and with each person and situation. It might seem as though we are on a roller coaster ride—up one day and down the next.

Don't be concerned about whether you are experiencing certain emotions or not. It is okay to feel happy as well as sad. It is okay to be angry when warranted. We may not always show our feelings to others even though we are experiencing them.

Resist the urge to compare yourself with others or judge how you are doing based on someone's opinion. This is especially important for husbands and wives who share a traumatic loss, such as the loss of a child, but have different styles and ways of facing it. Find a way to explain to the other what you are experiencing while accepting your differences in how you each express and handle your grief.

When moments of humor surface, we may think it will diminish our loss and grief. It doesn't. Cherish and welcome those moments. Laughter can offer that reprieve from the intensity of sorrow and depressive feelings that can settle over us like a heavy, suffocating cloak. We are not reducing or dismissing the importance of our loved one with humor or laughter.

Sometimes our grief can seem so overwhelming that we seek relief by throwing ourselves into a frenzy of activity. If we just keep busy enough, we think, we won't have time to feel. While activities certainly help us deal with our grief, activities by themselves will not take away our sorrow. We can anesthetize emotional pain for a while with drugs, liquor, denial, or activities; but eventually we are required to work through it.

Seek the assistance of a professional bereavement therapist or pastor when you are too overwhelmed to work on your own. It is important to get whatever assistance you need. Your life has been turned upside down. You have been hit a hard blow. Going through something like this is never easy, and we all need additional help and support.

Some things to consider:

1. Write down the emotions you are struggling with right now. Be specific. Expand your list. As emotions are identified, you will be able to work with them and through them.

2. Become aware of emotional patterns. Emotions will change from moment to moment and situation to situation. When we are out with friends, for example, life may seem normal. But when we return home, the walls close in and we become acutely aware of our loss once more. When do you experience grief more intensely? What new behaviors can you put in place in response to those times?

3. Read the Psalms. The Psalms speak to the human spirit in so many ways. Pray. Go through a meditation labyrinth. I found that when I walked on a nature trail or by the water, I was able to immerse myself in the timeless permanence of the world around me. It was healing to my soul. Painful thoughts and emotions were replaced with peace and serenity.

4. Establish soothing routines to put in place during difficult times of the day. Fix a cup of tea, play special music, call a friend. Post comforting and healing messages at various spots in your house to read as you walk past. Wrap yourself in a warm and soft quilt. Hug a fuzzy teddy bear. Put on soft and comfortable socks and clothes. Colors have an impact on our emotions. Replace dark, bright, or harsh colors with those that are more muted or pastel.

5. Treat yourself as you would a good friend. What would you do for a dear friend during such a time? Then do it for yourself. That is not being selfish. It is important.

6. Work on a meaningful project that will help redirect emotional energy from the sadness to something pleasant. It may be something you can do alone or with a group. Whatever it is, whether working with clay, coloring, painting, knitting, puttering in your workshop, quilting, hiking, or photography, make it a priority to do as often as possible.

   Think about it when you get up in the morning and imagine the enjoyment it will give you. If you are working full time, plan to do this at the end of the day or on weekends. If retired, choose some specific times. If possible, join a group who are doing similar things. This will give you the added benefit of connecting with others and creating a new circle of friends.

7. Start a gratitude book and begin writing down all the things you are grateful for, no matter how small or insignificant they may seem. Even the tiniest gratitude can heal a bruised and battered spirit. We are surrounded by blessings, but we often fail to recognize them unless we purposefully look for them. As we develop the skill of thankfulness, it will bring balance to the intensity of our grief.

8. Find supportive moments to talk with a trusted and compassionate friend about what you are experiencing. It is important to take time to share with another. Don't worry if your thoughts seem jumbled or disconnected. Sharing does not mean nonstop talking. Simple statements can reflect what you are experiencing. What is important is staying connected and being willing to accept offers of comfort and assistance. If you don't feel like talking, let your friends know in a gentle way that you can't talk right now, but that you really appreciate their care and compassion and would appreciate a listening ear another time.

CHAPTER 4

On Eagle's Wings— Let Go and Soar

"But they who wait for the LORD shall renew their strength,
they shall mount up with wings like eagles, they shall run and
not be weary, they shall walk and not faint."

ISAIAH 40:31

I'm tired—physically, emotionally, and spiritually. Grieving is harder than I could have imagined. Is there some magic formula that will make this easier? I'm tired of wandering the dark canyons and dry deserts of my soul. I'm tired of wondering when this will end.

There are days when I struggle to find a way into a new existence. How do I preserve what I had while letting go of what was? The memory of our love remains fresh in my mind, and I don't want to give it up.

Let go. Many times I have watched eagles from my deck, their powerful outstretched wings riding the thermal air currents, soaring upward until they were mere specks in the sky. How incredible to be an eagle serenely floating above my world and circumstances. But I can't soar if I hang on to what I had. I can't soar unless I release my grip of what I am clinging to.

Let go and soar. They say eagles mate for life; so did my husband and I. Like the pairs of eagles around my home, we worked and played together. Now, I am required to fly alone. But to be able to fly alone, I need to believe I can make it, to know that I will be okay by myself.

"In order to fly you have to let go of your fear and free fall, spreading your arms to catch the wind." It was something I had written in my journals months earlier as I was coming to terms with death while still hoping for a reprieve. Hope seemed like a double-edged sword cutting me to pieces. Yet without hope there is no purpose, no reason to believe in a future. "In order to fly, you must have hope. Hope can energize. Hope is the wings that will let me fly." I need to re-claim my own words for me today.

I close my eyes and become an eagle. As I liberate myself from the branches of past security and comfort, I feel my wings spreading, catching the invisible air currents of God's thermals. Rising higher and higher, I feel the ache in my heart and spirit melt away.

My mind focuses on the promises of God, confident that He will never leave me as I move out of the darkness of the unknown and into the light of new possibilities. When I need to fly, my wings will be strengthened. When I need to think and make the right decisions, my brain will become alert to see new opportunities. And waiting for me will be the thermal updrafts needed to soar above any state of affairs.

Let go and soar with the wings of an eagle—catch God's thermals and allow yourself to float on the security of God's love.

Reflection and Personal Application

How do you let go of a loved one and a life full of contentment and satisfaction? How do you pause in your grief to suspend the pain and sorrow and embrace a new life? One little step at a time.

Grieving a loss is never a straight line; there will be good days and bad days. There will be times when our energy is so depleted we struggle to get through the day; then there will be times when we feel energized.

The impact of bad days, however, can keep us from remembering the good days. Grieving often blinds us to anything that is positive.

Take some "time outs" while working through your loss in order to let go of sadness and soar above the grief. Relaxation and visualization enable us to do that. Relaxation begins with breathing slowly and evenly. Shallow breathing keeps us tense. Breathing that maintains good health comes from the diaphragm.

Here are ways to relax and use visualization

1. Find a quiet spot where you can sit comfortably and not be disturbed. If you have small children, be sure they are attended to. Close your eyes and start breathing deeply and evenly. Avoid shallow chest breathing. Instead, feel your diaphragm move in and out with each breath, as you breathe in through the nose and exhale slowly through the mouth. After you practice this a few times, you will notice your heart rate slowing to a steady and even rhythm and tension is being released from your muscles.

2. Relax your mind. Unless you are reminded of something urgent, such as the care and safety of your children, tell yourself you will attend to chores later; right now, your job is to relax. This is time out from activities. Do not resist or try to force thoughts away. This only increases tension. Instead, continue to breathe slowly and evenly and imagine your thoughts simply floating away. Then refocus on your breathing. Intruding thoughts can be very persistent and demanding. With practice, however, it becomes easier and easier to remain focused in the here and now. Continue to breathe in and out. Focus on different parts of your body where you hold tension. Breathe into these spots and let go of the tension as you breathe out.

3. After you are relaxed, extend and increase that relaxation with visualization. Our brain responds to pictures and symbols. Visualization is simply allowing your mind to produce positive mental images and pleasing pictures, either from old experiences

or new creations. These produce feelings of safety, deep tranquility and peace that will enhance healing of body and mind. When we are focused on hurtful and painful images, the opposite is true: we experience tension, anxiety, and helplessness.

Along with the positive mental pictures and images our brain produces, we are able to experience an entire range of sensory effects when deeply relaxed: the weightlessness of a soaring eagle or the warmth of a sandy beach. We can recall the smells of the ocean or pine forest or the sweet scent of flowers without any allergic reaction. Think back to times when you experienced peace and deep contentment; focus on these memories when you are relaxed.

4. Meditate on favorite Scripture verses of promise and comfort. Reflect on encouraging comments from others that have a relaxing effect on the mind and spirit.

5. When you have finished your relaxation and visualization exercise, count from three to one and open your eyes. Stretch your muscles and remain sitting for a few minutes before getting up for circulation to energize you again.

It does not take a long time to develop the habit of relaxing and calming deep breathing. And visualization is as easy as allowing your mind to rest on peaceful words and pictures of the mind. With experience you will be able to bring up that restful state whenever you close your eyes for a second, breathe deeply, and let go of tension.

CHAPTER 5

THAT STILL SMALL VOICE

"And there he came to a cave, and lodged there; and behold the
word of the LORD came to him, and he said to him, 'What are
you doing here, Elijah ... And behold, the LORD passed by, and
a great and strong wind rent the mountains, and broke in pieces
the rocks before the LORD, but the LORD was not in the wind;
and after the wind an earthquake, but the LORD was not in the
earthquake; and after the earthquake a fire; but the LORD was
not in the fire; and after the fire a still small voice."

1 KINGS 19:9, 11–12

In the depth of grief's despair and hopelessness, God comes and offers
me that one sentence in a book, that one word from a friend, that one
"aha!" moment that says *I have not left you. I have not abandoned you. I
do love you and am working things out for good in your life. Trust me, even
when you see no evidence for trust. Believe when there seems to be nothing
to believe.* That still small voice that moves mountains and calms the seas
reaches out and finds me in the darkest alleys or bright, neon-lit malls.

I repeat the words of the psalmist this morning: "God, you're my
last chance of the day; I spend the night on my knees. I've fallen in a
hole of oblivion. You've dropped me into a bottomless pit, sunk me in a

pitch-black abyss. I call to you, God; all day I call. I wring my hands and plead for help." And like Elijah, I crawl into my cave of depression and feel abandoned.

But I wasn't alone. God never left me. I picked up a book to read to escape the dreary morning clouds and listless feelings. Suddenly I heard that small but powerful voice booming in my ear. My heart jumped and burst into flame like a fire whose embers have been gently blown upon. Flames of hope ignited my spirit. Once more, my batteries were jump-started, and I felt resurgence of energy.

What an amazing thing! One moment I was listless, seeing no future, wanting only to remain in my comfortable chair beside the cozy fire, and then I am charged and ready to resume the dance of life. How does that happen?

There is power and spirit in words. Words spoken many centuries ago ring true over the ages. They contain within them the power to generate hope and peace and even joy. I'm in awe that there is a God who loves so much that He finds a way to reach us. That within those words there is this still small voice that breathes life into my life.

My heart is humbled, and I give quiet thanks.

Reflection and Personal Application

Support comes in many ways: words in a book, a phone call from a friend, Scripture, and stories I read. Grieving is not a journey to be completed in isolation, even though there are times when we want to be by ourselves. We need the encouragement, acceptance, and unconditional love of caring and compassionate people. We need to know we are not alone.

We help someone stay upright and stable by walking beside them as they go through the struggle. We can't take away another's pain, but we can let them know they are not alone. It was the willingness of my friends who listened and helped me ride the ups and downs of my grief journey over a long period of time that helped sustain me.

As grievers, we do not want to push our sadness onto others or burden them in any way. We don't want to intrude in the lives of our friends. There are times we just want to be alone, but there are other times when we want a consoling hug or listening ear. How do we convey this to others without appearing unappreciative or needy?

Friends may hesitate to reach out to us because they do not want to increase our pain by doing or saying the wrong thing. They want to help but are unsure in how to offer it. Should they continue to ask how we are doing when they see continued sadness? Or should they be silent and wait until the griever talks about what they are experiencing? Friends do not want to make it more difficult by offering assistance that may be misunderstood. So, they might retreat and do nothing.

How do we bridge this gap? As friends, we need the opportunity to offer support; as grievers, we need to receive it.

Some things to consider if you are grieving:

1. Give yourself permission to take whatever time is needed to recover and heal. It takes time for the layers of loss to be exposed. Each layer requires recognition and mourning. Resist the suggestions that you should be "over" your loss within a certain time frame.

2. Honor your way of doing things. While some people are emotionally expressive, others may find it difficult to say the words. Somewhere between the two extremes, we find ourselves struggling with words to express what is happening.

3. Share your doubts, questions, thoughts and anxieties about your future with a good friend and ask them to just listen; they don't have to give you advice or answers. Sharing helps put the pieces together when everything seems jagged and surreal. A good support group can be helpful as well as some sessions with a grief and loss counselor. When grief seems overwhelming, we begin to think there is something wrong with us. There is nothing wrong with you—you are in the very normal process of grieving.

4. Support doesn't always mean discussion. Working together on projects both you and your friend enjoy can allow the working out of grief. You can work in silence or talk about different things. Just being together is supportive. Healing can take place without words being spoken.

5. When friends ask you to dinner or want to include you in trips to the store, etc., say yes as often as possible, even if you don't feel like it. Pain can isolate us. Part of grieving is returning to the world we had known.

Appendix B at the back of this book offers more information about support.

CHAPTER 6

PRAYER

"Continue steadfastly in prayer,
being watchful in it with thanksgiving."

COLOSSIANS 4:2

E very morning I struggle to believe and trust. For forty-two years, I have awakened with my husband beside me. Now he is gone. There is an emptiness that fills the room, creating a void so deep I fear I will be swallowed up in its grasp. TV chatter and background music do nothing to fill that empty space.

My thoughts are scattered and jumbled, and I feel unsure about my future. What am I supposed to be doing? How do I find purpose and meaning for life again? God, you know the needs and wants of my heart, and I am sure you have a plan for me. But right now, the future looks as dark and empty as I feel.

Can our situations really be changed by praying? Do prayers actually make a difference? If there is a God and he is sovereign, doesn't he already know what the future holds and what I need? Why do I need to pray? Am I so desperate to get out of this state of mind that I am creating a false reality—an illusion of who God is? Yet, when I have looked for comfort and guidance throughout this grief and loss journey, verses that speak to the incredible heart of God have "jumped" out from the pages of my Bible, capturing my attention.

As I bring my doubts and pain to God, I have never felt a reprimand for any of my questioning, reservations, or insecurities. Instead, I am filled with a quiet hope and encouragement. Sometimes there is an immediate sense of peace after my urgent pleas; other times I receive clarity as I go about my day.

When I allow myself to think beyond the moment of desperation, I realize that my prayers are being heard and answered in so many ways: an instructive thought or confirmation after an internal struggle with uncertainties; an unexpected kind deed or encouraging word from a friend; strength to endure that came from something larger than myself. In those moments, I am also given the assurance that these things didn't just happen; that the God I believe in is a personal God who comforts and loves beyond what we can imagine.

Prayer to me is no longer some duty I must perform or a ritual or repetitious exercise. Instead, it is an ongoing conversation, an open-ended dialogue I have with God anytime, anywhere, and about anything. I can talk about my pain, needs, and wants. I can tell him when I feel angry about an unjust world, and when life is just too hard and unfair. I can be myself, exactly as I am: genuine, honest, and real in the moment. And I can wholeheartedly thank him for all the blessings I receive every day; the ability to work and laugh and cry and think and accomplish.

As I sit quietly, my internal dialogue has changed from one of despondency to a new measure of confidence. In the process, I no longer am ruled by conflicting thoughts and emotions. I am compelled to pick up my pen and paper and write about all the things I am learning, recording my progress. As I write, I feel my heart, soul, and spirit lifting.

Reflection and Personal Application

There is a spiritual as well as mental, psychological, and physical component to each of us. We will, regardless of faith or lack of it, be challenged by death as we come face-to-face with our own mortality, what we can and cannot do, and what we believe or don't believe.

Some might doubt there is a God, or if there is, that he does not have a personal interest in us. Others might feel we create myths to help us cope in moments of disaster or distress. Either way, when faced with death, loss, or trauma of any kind, our core beliefs will come under question.

This can be a positive time for spiritual and psychological growth. It can also be a time for discovery if you have wanted to believe in the past but could never reconcile your perceptions of what life and God should or ought to be. If you have had early experiences within a Christian church, but never felt connected, loss offers an opportunity to re-examine what your faith might be.

I cannot speak to non-Christian faiths or beliefs. The God I worship cares about us individually and collectively. It is a love I cannot earn or have to do ritualistic penance to receive. It is a love that is freely given to any who humbly want to receive it. As we are confronted with death, it is an opportunity to explore what life and death mean and gain a more meaningful appreciation for both.

If you struggle with the concept of a God or a spiritual side, you might find healing more difficult. We do heal, and we do survive. But it was faith and belief that enabled me to find both purpose and meaning again on a personal level. It was prayers, both mine and those of others, along with faith that brought me to a deeper understanding of God and myself.

In our despondency and misery, the need for pain to end can become so tremendous that we plead for immediate relief. We are like the man in the desert dying from thirst. When given water, he gulps it down and quickly holds out his cup for more. In our desire to return to a world of stability and certainty, we try to gulp down enough comfort, hope, and peace to make it happen right away. At times it seems as though we have holes in our cups and the well-being we crave drains out as fast as it is poured in.

So, it is with our requests. "God fix me. Give me that shot of spiritual morphine to deaden this pain—that elixir of life to make everything okay again." And we want it now, not in the future. But there is a progression from wounding to healing in human time. Throughout the course of crying out, I have found God working in his timing. As I synchronize my own needs with that timing, I have been given the strength, resiliency, and peace to meet the challenges I come against.

So, do prayers make a difference? There is scientific and medical evidence that show prayers make a difference in healing from surgeries and injuries, regardless of whether the recipient knows he is being prayed for or not. My training is rooted in science, and I find many direct correlations between science and the Word of God. While Scripture gives us the information we need to live moral lives, the science of psychology gives us tools to apply that information.

It is easy to get discouraged. When we feel no relief, it may seem as though our requests and questions remain unanswered. Is there really a God? Does he hear us? Does he care? Why don't I feel better? Like most of us, I wanted an immediate response to my questions. But healing takes time. I discovered, when I left my pain and depressed spirit with God each morning and resumed my daily routines, answers were given.

Grieving could be likened to an athlete who works out every day to develop the strength and skills required to compete. Both take both time and energy; it's hard work. And with both there will be many days we do not see progress.

Spiritual muscles also require a daily workout that begins with a small spark of faith and hope and continues with some kind of action each day. Spiritual development begins when we spend time with God, prayer and the Word of God. As with physical development, there will be days when we see little progress in our spiritual development. But as we persevere, not only is our faith strengthened, but our sphere of understanding and hope expanded, our pain diminished, and our pervasive sadness begins to fade.

My idea of prayer may be different than yours. For me, it no longer is a religious duty or ritual, but a relationship I treasure. It is a part of my internal dialogue—that streaming of consciousness that occurs all the time. Just as in other close relationships, sometimes there is a volume of words. Other times, no words need to be spoken; the spirit says it all—and it is simply understood by our friend.

Whether or not you have a belief, you can explore this concept by simply starting a conversation. You may have been afraid to talk with God in the past. But Scripture tells us over and over again that he loves us, and we are encouraged to draw near to him with honesty and humility.

Here are some ways to start that dialogue. Close your eyes and imagine you are talking with your closest friend. A trusted and loyal friend allows you the freedom and safety to discuss anything without fear of being rejected or reprimanded. Now see God as this friend who cares about you and has your best interests at heart.

1. What would you like to say to God if he were sitting in the chair in front of you? For example: *Why did this have to happen? Why me? Do You really love me? Do You really care?* Tell Him about your doubts and uncertainties. Start an honest conversation that shares your hurts, needs, and concerns. Be willing to listen.

2. Tell God if you feel angry. Sometimes we are afraid to talk to God about our anger directly. He already knows your pain and your anger. Speak it. Be honest.

3. What worries and concerns would you like to ask God to help you with? For example: *Finances; managing a home without the person I loved. Or perhaps, why should I believe.*

4. Ask for clarification and for enough faith to wait for answers. Ask for help to trust even when answers aren't imminent.

5. Make a list of all the times your prayers have been answered in the past, even if they were simple exclamations of "God help me!" Reflect on those prayers and answers you received, even if you hadn't considered them answers at the time.

6. Explore the Book of Psalms in the Bible to discover more about the character of God.

CHAPTER 7

AND GOD SAID, "REST"

"O that I had wings like a dove! I would fly away and be at rest."

PSALM 55:6

A Scripture I heard at church recently that indicated that God disciplines his children for their good. I thought, "Am I being disciplined for some reason? What am I supposed to be learning and doing in this valley of sorrow?"

But then, I heard God's quiet but powerful voice say to me, "Rest—you are learning to rest. You are not to do anything or try to make anything happen. Just rest."

Rest? What does that mean? How do I take it easy in the midst of all this mental and emotional turmoil? How can I relax in this journey through my desert of dried up old bones where dreams and plans about life have crumbled into dust? I can keep busy or divert my attention with books or TV, but that is only a temporary distraction. Grieving a loss while creating a new life is more than just keeping busy or diverting the mind so we don't feel; it is processing and integrating what has happened.

When I was a young housewife, my days were filled with juggling schedules of three children (two with special needs) and a husband who worked several jobs. I got a break when I could finish folding the laundry without disturbance or do some creative sewing or work in the garden without worrying about what my kids were getting into. Later, when I went back to work and then onto school to complete college degrees, my schedule was even more complex and demanding. Relaxation came when I could study for class instead of cleaning the house. Even quick day trips away with my husband were often filled with activities, giving only temporary reprieve from the pressure of ongoing life and work.

If "rest" simply becomes another item on our to-do list, it will become another "have to" or stressor instead. Rest is more than taking a quick break from chores or schedules. It is finding quiet time where healing can occur.

When I choose to rest, I sit quietly, close my eyes, and see myself as a little child. I feel the strong and tender arms of God's spirit surround me, and I hear his words of assurance. I let go of the stress, uncertainties, pain, and loneliness that keep collecting. Gradually, my muscles release their tension, my mind focuses on relaxing, and my breathing becomes steady and even. There is no need to ask for anything. I can just "be." My mind and spirit become quiet and still.

And I rest.

Reflection and Personal Application

The world does not stop while we recover from our drastically altered reality. We are required to continue with jobs, take care of children, pay our bills, and basically resume all the normal daily activities of life. As we do, we make the assumption that we have no more time to grieve; it's time to move on.

After a while, we may be tempted to box in the remaining troubling questions and passionate emotions and ignore their presence. Sometimes we just want it all to be over and we block them off. It is easier "not to feel" than work through ongoing emotions and avoid working through unanswered questions. Maybe if we ignore them, they will just all go away and we can find rest.

But they don't go away. It requires energy and willpower to keep unprocessed tragedies and distressing grief locked up and restrained.

Research on Post Traumatic Stress Disorder (PTSD) has shown that repressed traumatic events, along with their emotions and thoughts, do not just go away. Much of a therapist's work is helping individuals uncover, release and heal from unpleasant and painful events in the past. When we come to terms with our losses, reconcile the conflicts, and end the mental struggles, we are able to let go and grieve. We are able to "feel" again.

Throughout life, it is essential to take time for rest and reflection where we can allow our spirits to rise above the mundane. In those moments, our minds and spirits become renewed and our perception of self, others, and God are expanded. This is especially important when grieving.

During this time period, find moments within the demands of each day to rest. Grieving requires more time than just a few weeks, months or even a year. The serious business of working through the knots and tangles associated with our endings often do not begin until after those initial days and months. We need those quiet, reflective and restful moments to integrate dangling and frayed pieces of our past into a new cohesive life structure.

Here are some suggestions about resting:

1. Find quiet time outside your busy schedule to connect with the enduring stability and beauty of nature. Walk on the beach or on a wooded trail. Immerse yourself in these surroundings. There is symmetry, harmony, and order in nature. Stop to observe more closely the intricate beauty of a flower or the hum of a bumblebee. Even if you are not an outdoors person, these can be incredibly healing moments. I spent many moments on my deck during the early days of my grieving, where I simply absorbed the beauty of blooming flowers, felt the sun on my skin, and listened to the variety of birds sing and the whir of hummingbirds coming for their morning sips of nectar. Time seemed suspended. Such instances take us out of our fast-paced

existence and allow us to be in the moment. Experiencing and engaging in the beauty of nature can be extremely therapeutic.

2. Reflect on those times in the past when you were doing something you really enjoyed. Perhaps it was gardening or painting or building something. Maybe you lost yourself in knitting or quilting, or rearranging furniture to create beauty and comfort in your home. Interest in people and places may have generated happy hours of making travel plans; time was suspended, and you were unaware of hours passing. Whatever the project, it gave you satisfaction, pleasure, and contentment. Can you begin doing some of those things again?

3. Practice being in the moment. Here are some suggestions:

   • Listen to music you enjoyed in the past. Allow the melodic sounds and pleasing tones to become a comforting blanket, releasing tension and soothing each nerve and cell in the body. Imagine each note is like the downiest feather from your softest down quilt absorbing pain and relaxing the fibers of your mind and body. Breathe and relax deeply into these healing images.

   • Watch young children play. Children by nature are free and uninhibited. Remember the times when you were engrossed in play as a child, your mind completely absorbed with discovery and imagination. Experience that again.

   • Observe the activities of nature: the busyness of bees, the patience of a spider on his web, or the industry of insects. They overcome great obstacles and accomplish great feats.

4. Absorb yourself in the here and now as you observe life around you. There are no clocks or time —only the present; the past and future are irrelevant. For a few minutes just *exist*. Expand those moments whenever you can.

5. Using the relaxation techniques described in Chapter Four, relax and create healing and quieting visualizations. Our brain responds to symbols and pictures. Relaxation, meditation and visualization have been successfully used to manage physical pain and reduce stress in the medical community. It is also beneficial for healing and reducing emotional and psychological pain. Some healing images for healing the mind and body can be as simple as visualizing yourself lying in a warm, soothing pool of water. As you relax, feel tension and pain melt away.

6. Create other visualizations that are peaceful and restful that will also have a direct mind and body response. It might be walking through a meadow, breathing in the clean smells of a forest or connecting to the pulse of the gentle rolling surf. Allow your mind to bring up its own restful scenes that incorporate all the senses.

7. Rest is anything that takes you out of the "have to" world and gives you permission to do nothing for short periods of time. It allows our mind and body to recover, heal and re-charge.

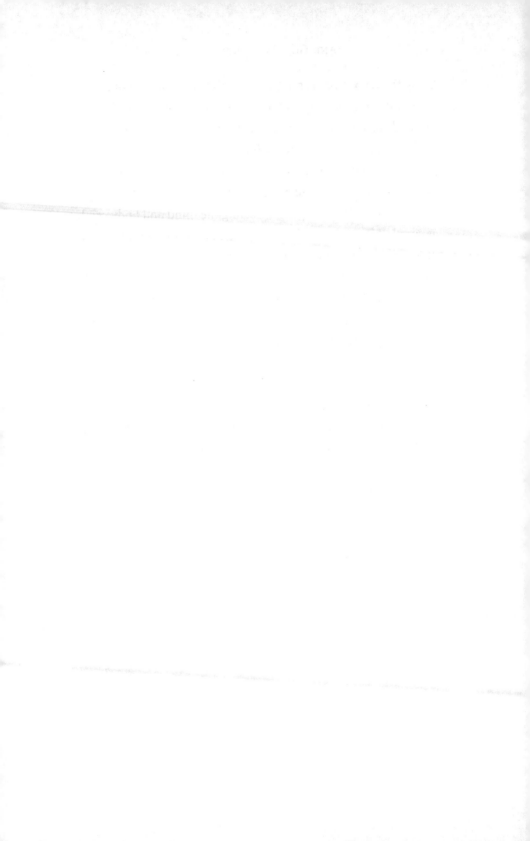

PART II
LETTING GO;
CLOSING THE DOOR

CHAPTER 8

BATTLES

"God, God, save me! I'm in over my head ... I'm hoarse from calling for help, bleary-eyed from searching the sky for God ... Pull me out of the clutch of the enemy. This whirlpool is sucking me down ... Now answer me God, because you love me. Let me see your great mercy full-face. Don't look the other way; your servant can't take it. I'm in trouble. Answer right now ... Come close, God; get me out of here. Rescue me from this deathtrap."

PSALM 69:1, 3; 16; 18–20 *THE MESSAGE*

As I read and prayed the psalms this morning, I realized I was still on the front lines of a battle and the enemy was loneliness and depression. I struggle to create a new meaningful life. Like the psalmist, I identify with the whirlpool that wants to suck me down. And like him, I too cry out for rescue.

Looking for assurance, I flipped the pages of my Bible. It opened to the gospel of Matthew. In chapter nine, I read the story of Jesus and two blind men. They came to him begging to be healed. They too wanted to be saved from their life of despair. Jesus asked them if they believed he could heal them. When they answered yes, Jesus then responded, "Become what you believe."

This same chapter in Matthew contained two other stories that had an impact on me this morning. A local official approached Jesus and told Jesus his daughter had just died; but if Jesus would just come and touch her, she would live. On the way to this man's house, a woman reached out from the crowd and touched the hem of Jesus' robe. "If I could just put a finger on his robe," she thought, "I would get well. " Jesus felt that touch, stopped, turned, and reassured her with these words, "Courage, daughter. You took a risk of faith and now you're well."

Become ... believe ... courage ... faith ... risk ...

As I read and write these words, I feel them speaking to me, "Courage, Marlene. Take that risk of faith. Continue to follow God. He will fill your life with purpose and meaning again, and you will become what you believe."

How do we get from here to there? How do we get courage? How does our faith turn into action? By making tough choices and taking baby steps until our legs get strong enough to walk with confidence. Courage is developed little by little as we step out in faith toward a new reality.

Reflection and Personal Application

When a favorite comforter has been torn, there is a huge gap that no longer covers us with warmth and comfort. Even when we try to adjust the blanket around us, the hole is too big and the cold comes in.

Our losses are a huge tear in the fabric of our lives. Until that fabric is re-woven, there will be gaps leaving us exposed and feeling defenseless to life's battles and challenges. We will get discouraged, overwhelmed and sometimes disheartened as we struggle to find new meaning and purpose for our lives again.

Depression and loneliness are often two unwanted travelers that we do battle with. Loneliness occurs when we feel isolated from others because of the great change that has occurred. Loss shifts the normal patterns of life and relationships.

If you lost a spouse, the social activities you shared with other couples have now changed. As a single person, your identity within those social circles is different. The dynamics and commonalities are no longer the same. There are triangles instead of foursomes. We struggle to develop new social structures.

If your loss was a child or long-awaited child, you no longer fit within the conversations of parents who share the joys and concerns of parenting. If disease or an accident has disabled you from doing the routine things you once enjoyed with others, your association within those same circles will gradually become more difficult. This is another layer of loss that requires new ways to connect with people in new social settings.

All losses strip us of who we were before. The patterns of living and routines that we accepted as normal have now been altered. We are not just taking back our life; we are finding new ways to define that life.

Some losses and their accompanying layers will require a greater adjustment than others. In the struggle to accommodate new roles, we may experience uncertainty, hesitation and doubt. Pervasive feelings of inadequacy and discouragement can become the norm if we allow them to become a habit.

It is normal and natural to experience periods of loneliness and depression when grieving. There will be bad days. Your normal pattern of living and doing things has been drastically altered, creating doubts and uncertainty about your future. Everything comes in question: your dreams, goals, and purpose – everything. Recognizing that this can happen can help us put it into a different perspective. While they can become obstacles for a short period of time as we adjust to a new way of life, they do not need to become permanent or long-lasting roadblocks.

If you have a history of depression, you may want to seek out a good professional therapist, preferably one familiar with cognitive behavioral strategies. Sometimes medication is needed to help us through a tough period. But reframing the things you say to yourself about what is happening can make a huge difference. Instead of saying, I will never be happy again, tell yourself you are finding new ways to bring happiness into your life.

Here are some other self-help strategies you can apply that are very beneficial. They can help reduce depression.

1. Establish schedules and routines. They can be altered later as needed. Chaotic surroundings can feed anxiety and depression. Routines establish normalcy and stability. Have regular mealtimes and eat something even when you aren't hungry. Include some form of exercise every day, whether it is going for a short or extended walk.

2. Maintain regular sleep habits. Sleep allows the body and mind to heal. Get up and go to bed at a regular time, even if you don't feel sleepy. Sleep is often disturbed because our minds focus on our losses during that time of day. Allow this routine to guide you back into a normal sleep pattern. If you wake up in the night, put a low light on and read a book. Some people suggest actually getting out of bed to read and then returning to bed when you get sleepy. I have found it easier to read in bed. Sometimes a cracker or warm milk can help.

3. Examine your overall patterns of activity. Which ones give you satisfaction or joy? Which drain you of energy and becomes yet another burden to endure? What activities are only diversions to avoid what we are feeling? Can you redirect your energy to activities that energize you or make you feel good?

4. Sometimes words aren't enough to articulate what we are experiencing; we need other forms of artistic endeavors that can reach into that dimension where there are no words, just the heart and soul giving expression to what we are feeling. This is a project just for you even if you do it within a group. This is you expressing your love, joy, sorrow, frustration, anger, and tears; it is not doing to please someone else. This is you telling your story within a wall hanging or collage or sculpted lump of clay. This is you communicating love, yearning and sorrow as you put together the pieces of what you held dear. Find an

art therapy class if you are unsure where to begin or take some other beginning art class. Or just work on your own. Mold clay. Cut and paste collages. Sew bits and pieces together. Explore options and then use whatever medium draws your heart and soul.

5. Volunteer some time at a local hospital or agency. Losing a loved one can make us feel we are no longer valued or needed. Even with a full-time job, doing volunteer work on the weekends can be healing. Find someone or something to devote time and energy.

6. Avoid relying on drugs or alcohol to make you feel better. They simply create a new set of problems. If munchies help you through the long evenings, eat foods that are healthy and limit their intake. The simple pleasure of eating food can be comforting; but it can create other types of problems.

CHAPTER 9

BLESSED ARE THE POOR IN SPIRIT

"Blessed are the poor in spirit,
for theirs is the kingdom of heaven."

MATTHEW 5:3

I was asked once if I thought the only way we would discover God was through pain or loss. I've thought a lot about that. Surely it doesn't take tragedies to experience God. And yet, I think perhaps it does. Maybe it's only when we are overwhelmed, broken, and "poor in spirit" that we are ready to acknowledge a need for someone greater than ourselves.

We are physically born in pain. And perhaps that is the only way we can be born spiritually as well. Pain wears many faces: the pain of loss, emptiness, and disillusionment; the pain of guilt and shame, rejection, and abandonment. Within all pain we find ourselves struggling to find answers.

We search for meaning in academic institutions and in the wisdom of philosophers. We believe we will be happy when we have reached a certain level of success or have acquired enough wealth. We make plans, work hard to achieve them, and believe we are good people because we attend church each week. Yet in all our endeavors, do we actually "experience" God?

I don't believe we will find him in lofty academic institutions (although he wants us to educate, develop, and use our minds). We won't find him in the rich man's house or amongst our treasures (although he doesn't begrudge us riches or wealth). I believe we only find him when we don't have the answers and can't even formulate the questions; when our well-laid plans have been destroyed and we are stripped of wealth, good intentions, and well-designed lives.

What a marvelous and mysterious God we have. He patiently waits for us to respond to his invitation to walk with him; an invitation we rarely see until faced with tragedy. Then when we reach out and take his extended hand, we are able to experience his love and compassion. Our spirits are lifted, our resolve is strengthened, and we see with "new eyes."

And it is with the "new eyes" of a spirit blessed by God where we are enriched by all he has designed. The breathtaking sunset and inviting sunrise with skies painted shades of pink and red, yellow and orange take on a new depth and beauty. We not only see the fragility of delicate flowers and flitting butterflies but also see their strength and resiliency. The intricate designs on the beaches shaped by wind and waves formed with carefree abandon become major works of art.

I have witnessed hurricanes and tornados as they rip across the landscape. I have been engulfed by the quiet, deadly fog that rolls in, catching mariners by surprise. I am humbled by the awesome power of an Almighty God. And my spirit is blessed because I am a part of his plan.

Reflection and Personal Application

The University of Life hands us some tough assignments. When those life assignments are filled with pain, we will do anything and everything to get rid of it as quickly as possible. We try to escape in some way by deadening it with alcohol, prescription drugs, food, or endless activity; anything just so we don't have to feel and can avoid addressing it.

While we may hate pain, it has a purpose. It protects and helps us survive by telling us what isn't right that we need to pay attention to. That is true for both physical and emotional or psychological pain. It enables us to make necessary corrections. Pain lets us know if we need to change directions, slow down, or take a time out from life so we can examine more constructive ways to live.

Psychological and emotional pain can teach us valuable lessons that will enrich our lives such as what is truly important in the long run. Pain forces me to stop and reflect on what is working and what is not working. When I allow myself to learn from it, I can see and accept my vulnerabilities, break down the protective and limiting barriers I have built, and allow my pain to strengthen me instead of disabling me. It is within its time and space that I can become real, honest and genuine.

Some things to consider:

1. What valuable lessons are you learning from your pain during this time period?
2. What face is your pain wearing today? Is it the face of guilt, anger, rejection, bitterness, deep sorrow, or depression? Sit with it awhile. Don't try to alter or change how you feel. Simply sit with your pain and tell it you are listening. Write down the valuable insights you receive.
3. Write down the things you are learning about yourself, your world, and God through your hurts and sorrows. You are much more than your pain or your losses. As we give ourselves permission to work through our anguish, it gradually loses its grip on us.

CHAPTER 10

LET GOD LEAD

"Therefore, do not be anxious, saying, 'What shall we eat?' or
'What shall we drink?' or 'What shall we wear?' For the Gentiles
seek all these things; and your heavenly Father knows that you
need them all. But seek first his kingdom and his righteousness,
and all these things shall be yours as well. Therefore, do not be
anxious about tomorrow, for tomorrow will be anxious for itself.
Let the day's own trouble be sufficient for the day."

MATTHEW 6:31–34

I find no comfort in these words this morning. In fact, I want to start
building sturdy walls around my heart to shut out any and all emotions. I am tired of feeling sad and am exhausted from crying. If I am
going to survive, I'm going to have to do it by myself without any help
from God or anyone else.

But there was no escape from that unrelenting emptiness and appre-
hension that persisted in spite of my angry, strong-willed determination.
I really do need those words of comfort, encouragement, and motivation
I get each morning from Scripture. Throughout this journey, whenever
I have opened my Bible, passages that I needed for that day would stand

out as if highlighted in neon lights. They were passages of God's love and care that I desperately needed to rebuild my life.

Getting over my funk, I sit down and randomly open my Bible. It opens to the thirtieth chapter of Jeremiah, and I started to read. "Don't despair, Israel ... The time is coming when I will turn everything around for my people, both Israel and Judah. I, God, say so." It seemed those words were being spoken to me: "Don't despair, Marlene. The time is coming, when I will turn things around in your life."

While I can bulldoze my way through this grief, get angry, deny my feelings of sadness, and even build protective walls around my heart, at some point I will have to deal with both my emotions and the thoughts that created them. Negative thoughts can't just be pushed away or ignored; they need to be acknowledged, challenged, and replaced.

Reflection and Personal Application

The grief and loss journey is never straightforward—it goes up and down and often takes many detours. It can be likened to a trip we make across country in our car. The road can take us up steep mountain passes with hairpin turns and then plunge back down into deep, narrow canyons with steep walls that block the light. There will be rest stops and points of interest to explore.

As we climb, plateaus and breathtaking panoramas will be revealed. We may experience threatening dark clouds and storms, sheets of rain that pelt us like tiny needles. Bright sunshine coloring the landscape with rich colors will tease our senses. There will be roads of barren desert that stretch endlessly before us with hot burning sand, dotted with inhospitable cacti and monstrous distorted rocks rising from nowhere.

Grieving will take us up and down these rocky paths hard to traverse and into dark, foreboding canyons that block the light of hope. There will be dry, barren periods that seem to go on forever with no nourishment for our spirits. Sometimes it may seem we have entered a world hit by a cataclysmic earthquake that leaves huge, jagged and threatening upheavals, obstacles that keep us from going anywhere.

It is natural to want this journey to end and want to resume a life that holds the potential for happiness and contentment again. We want to experience once more the natural relaxed ease of living. And just when we think we can't go any further, we discover we have climbed new heights of understanding that holds within its grasp unlimited possibility; reaching new vistas of opportunity.

While we may want to hurry things along, some things cannot be rushed. Looking for an easy solution such as walling off emotions or getting angry without tempering it with rational thought may not bring the results we want. For me, God was a steadying force, allowing the healing process to move forward in its own timely manner. When I tried to change that timing, I only made it more difficult. It was a lesson in patience I needed to learn.

Because anger is often an emotion that can hamper our progress, I have chosen to address it within this chapter. Other intense emotions, such as guilt and shame, are also part of that mix of complex emotions that can impede the healing progress and prolong the working out of grief. I have added additional information about these emotions at the end of this book in Appendix A.

If your loss was unexpected or the result of an injustice or someone's irresponsible behavior anger may become problematic. What happened was unfair and makes no sense; and we grapple with the conflict it creates. It crashes into our sense of order and justice and reasonable expectations. Anger can be triggered over and over again making it difficult to work through our grief unless we address it.

Here are some things to consider about anger:

1. Recognize and acknowledge your anger. Do not deny or push it away. It will only resurface and get worse, resulting in bitterness and resentment. While anger is a normal and natural reaction to unfair and unjust circumstances, what is important is what we

do with that anger. Anger as other emotional responses depends on how we perceive a situation. We are responsible for it and can intensify its effect on us. Step back and think more rationally about its importance to us.

2. Find a healthy way to release the immediate tension of anger. Pound a pillow; go to the gym and work out. Run. Walk. Move until the anger energy is released or reduced. But remember, that while we are releasing anger energy, the source of the anger is still there and needs to be addressed. Cooling off allows us to think and place events into a larger context.

3. Resist the temptation to seek revenge or harbor a grievance; it only allows the anger and pain to thrive and grow. Anger has a purpose. It can help us survive and serve as a motivation to make changes and new positive goals. It is our responsibility to choose what we do with our anger. Resentments and grievances are self-destructive.

4. Write about your anger. What is it telling you? What can you learn from it? Be completely honest. Research has shown that writing helps to tone down the intensity of our anger and helps clarify what it means to us. Keep writing until you see a larger picture. There are many constructive ways to grieve that will bring about the healing you desire. If you have had an ongoing anger problem, please seek professional counseling to help work through the causes associated with it.

CHAPTER 11

ACCEPTANCE

"Why are you down in the dumps, dear soul? Why are you crying the blues? Fix my eyes on God—soon I'll be praising again. He puts a smile on my face. He's my God."

PSALM 43:5 *THE MESSAGE*

Acceptance this morning does not feel like a promise of a new beginning. Instead, it is a bitter pill added to the string of losses I have been asked to accept: my husband, my home, retirement, my daughter's cancer, a degenerating hip ...

Mornings are the hardest. There could have been so many more years with my husband. My mind struggles with recurring doubts and misgivings. God, why is this so hard? Will I ever find a sense of contentment and sustained peace once more? Every day I cry out to you. Isn't it time to leave this barren wasteland that stretches on forever?

And I can't help asking: *God, do you really care about us personally? Do you want us to be happy?* But even as I think it, I know the answer. He does care. If he didn't, the Bible would simply be another piece of idealistic literature created by man, and the God we believe in would either be nonexistent or a God of cruel proportions as he teased us with words of love while destroying us with indifference and impossible demands.

When I stepped out onto my deck early this morning with my coffee, notebook, and Bible, I reflected again on the life I had with my husband. Ours was a close and dependable relationship. Words were often not required; flowers not needed. An endearing note signed by a drawn paw-print of our little dog spoke volumes.

It seemed we fit like a hand and glove. We knew each other's thoughts without speaking; seeking and holding hands without conscious thought, an unspoken understanding of each other's needs. We accepted the quirks of each other; didn't allow trivialities to interfere and could laugh at our own foibles and with each other. Now, waking up alone after a lifetime together with someone I loved, it is difficult to move forward.

As a therapist, I know that acceptance is the first step in letting go of the past in order to see new choices. But my mind and spirit do not want to let go of the life I had. Although I am grateful for all those wonderful years, waking up alone is still very difficult.

Every morning I turn to and am comforted by God's promises. However, doubts can quickly come and rob me of that peace as I go about my day. I know God cares, yet when the future seems uncertain and bleak it is easy to forget.

I pick up my Bible and read again from the Psalms. Once again my doubts are replaced with quiet assurance that God is always there with me and will give me the strength and wisdom I need each day.

A veiled sun warms me as I sit quietly on my deck and reflect. As the clouds dissipate, I feel God's Spirit dispelling the mists of questions and uncertainty, and I no longer feel alone. God is working "for good" through all of this, even when I am unaware of it. It is a quiet work that gradually transforms my life from one of grief and sorrow to one of possibility and new beginnings.

Reflection and Personal Application

Acceptance and letting go is a process that begins with a conscious choice. We stop fighting the reality we don't want and make a shift in our thinking. It is an ongoing purposeful determination.

There is a natural resistance to accept the ending of something that was important and valuable to us. Drastic change of any kind is hard. When the change comes from the loss of what you loved and valued the most, it becomes even more difficult to accept and reconcile. Letting go of what we loved, however, does not diminish that love we valued.

Within acceptance, we come to terms with what has happened: no more denials, resistance or wishful thinking; we make a conscious decision to end the conflict of unanswered questions, confusion and doubts and stop fighting with God, self and others. Life isn't fair and we will never have all the answers we want. We still grieve but are freed from becoming perpetual prisoners to that grief. It is where reconciliation begins as we choose to believe that something good will come from all of this.

Acceptance is not the end – it is the beginning. It isn't giving up. Rather, it is a conscious option to leave the past in the past. We give ourselves permission to live again as we take the ashes of our tragedies and begin creating something new and positive. Intense emotions are neutralized, and we experience peace and calm.

When we come to the edge of a cliff with only desolation behind us, we may feel our options are limited. But if we remain in the ruins of what was, we will not be able to build a bridge to cross the chasm of uncertainty and begin looking for new opportunities. Acceptance and letting go releases our energy to build that bridge.

Integrating our losses occurs over time. It may seem at times as though we are making no progress. But positive change is happening. We may be required to make that choice of acceptance more than once as we step out in faith.

Some questions to consider:

1. Where are you in your grief process? What layers associated with your loss have been recognized? Take time to grieve and come to terms with each of them.
2. What part of your loss do you find difficult to accept and continue to struggle with? Can you take that first baby step and

release it? Tuck it safely in your memories. It is not gone. You can revisit it at any time.

3. What important elements of the past are you taking with you as you move forward? Perhaps it is a special way of doing things that was shared with your loved one. Some people return to favorite places or make that trip that couldn't be completed before. Sometimes we find ourselves integrating ideals and principles that held importance. I find myself seeing and responding more to the humorous side of life as my husband did. It is okay to hold onto something tangible that had great importance in the life of your deceased. These can be strengthening and loving remembrances that you take with you and apply to your life today.

CHAPTER 12

THE STRUGGLE TO BELIEVE

"God, are you avoiding me? Where are you when I need you?"

PSALM 10:1 *THE MESSAGE*

"Long enough, God—you've ignored me long enough. I've looked at the back of your head long enough. Long enough I've carried this ton of trouble, lived with a stomach full of pain."

PSALM 13:1–2 *THE MESSAGE*

God, are you ignoring me? Are you there? It seems like ages since I have felt your presence. Although I am moving forward, I wake up to an empty house and a pervasive loneliness. I read your Word and ponder the cries of those who came before me. And like them, I cry out, "Hear my prayers, Lord. Help me through this unwanted journey!"

Mornings and evenings remain the hardest times of the day as I struggle to come to terms with this new reality. During the day, work and friends occupy my mind. But when I return home, tired in body and spirit, the realization sinks in once more that I do not have anyone waiting to share the trivialities of the day. I fix my plate of warmed-up food and put the TV on for company. Even the surreal world of TV hype and glitter is better than the all-encompassing world of silence.

Why is it so hard to survive? At times, I feel as though I am on a battlefield. Life is full of struggles. We struggle to pay the bills, to survive disappointments, and to resolve conflicts. We struggle to be heard, seen, accepted, and loved. We harden our hearts and build protective walls so we don't have to feel any more pain when we are rejected.

Perhaps it is only within such wrestling where we find purpose and meaning for life. As we work through the uncertainties, losses, and despairs, we discover ourselves and develop the spiritual and emotional muscles to persevere, grow strong, and become resilient.

When everything goes well, we are autonomous and independent and forget the necessity for God and others. But when pain, anxiety, and fear hold us in their grips, we realize our desperate need for sovereignty beyond ourselves. It is where; if we are willing to turn to God, we will find him ready to help. Then in those moments of desperation, we are able to celebrate our rescue and sing like the psalmist in Psalm 98, "Sing to God a brand-new song. He's made a world of wonders!"

Reflection and Personal Application

Questions surface as we work through the tangled remains of endings. Besides the usual legal necessities of changing titles to homes and cars, the loss of a spouse can raise many questions such as: What do I do now? Should I move or stay where I am?

If you lost your spouse through divorce, the questions may be similar, but they take on the added dimension of anger and betrayal. When there are small children, their welfare becomes a crucial part of decision making. If you lost a favored grandparent or best friend with whom you could talk about anything, your question might be: Now who can I talk to about my doubts and fears and uncertainties?

Each loss will present its own special and unique set of circumstances and conditions. Each person, within his or her individual personality and life experiences, will be challenged with questions pertinent to their unique situation. A couple may grieve the loss of their child differently from one another. Time of death, depth of emotional attachment, and personal expectations will influence the intensity of our grief and the ability to come to terms with it. The loss of an aging grandparent who we do not want to see suffer will create a different response to our grief process than one who is still vibrant and full of life.

Starting over can seem ominous and intimidating. You may struggle to believe that you can and will make it. During this time period, resist making any drastic lifestyle changes that are not necessary. Hasty decisions based on the emotions of the moment can create future problems. If we make quick decisions hoping to end our grief or believe that it will relieve our sadness, it may not provide the relief we want. Emotions are worked through, so our decision making is connected with conscious choices to move toward something new rather than escape from what we don't want.

As you seek answers to important life decisions, friends may not be the best choice to offer realistic or honest advice because of their desire to be protective of our emotional state. Seek the counsel of people you respect and who are knowledgeable about similar circumstances. Tell them exactly why you are wrestling with the problem you are facing and ask for both the benefits and risks involved with all options. Be willing to pay for a consultation, if necessary, to get the best expert advice available to you.

We never have all the facts and data we need in our decision making. There will always be unknowns. But if you have collected as much available information as possible, you will be able to carefully weigh the pros and cons and make a good informed decision. Pray for wisdom and guidance throughout the process. Trust in your ability to make decisions that are right for you.

Ask yourself the following questions:

1. What decision am I facing right now? Does it involve a major move, a new career, resolving financial concerns, etc.?
2. On a sheet of paper, list each problem, potential options, and the risks and benefits involved. Do I need additional information from qualified people? Who can help me?

3. Resist making drastic or life-altering changes as you readjust and regain your balance, such as a major home move. Ask yourself, do I really need to make this move right now? What are the costs and benefits of staying where I am? Current wisdom dictates waiting at least a year.

4. Am I using emotions to influence my decision-making process instead of reasoning through the pros and cons connected with each of my options? If so, take some additional time to reconcile or resolve feelings so you can make a good choice based on reason and logic.

CHAPTER 13

A Time to Laugh and a Time to Cry

"For everything there is a season, and a time for every matter
under heaven: a time to be born, and a time to die; a time to
plant, and a time to pluck up what is planted; a time to kill,
and a time to heal; A time to break down, and a time
to build up; a time to weep, and a time to laugh;
a time to mourn, and a time to dance."

ECCLESIASTES 3:1–4

A time to laugh and another to cry—a time to live and a time to die.
This has been my time to weep and mourn and be in solitude; a
time to retreat, find my soul, and recover my spirit from the depths of my
sorrow. It has been a period to be alone and find rest from the exertion
of wanting so desperately to find contentment again. But maybe more
importantly, it has been a time to reflect and be grateful for all I have been
given; and then cut my losses and let go. I crave peace in my acceptance.

I want to change this season of weeping to one of laughter and contentment. Am I ready to let go of what was in order to reach out to a new

tomorrow that may be radically different from what I had before? My heart says, "Yes, I want to laugh and sing and dance. I'm tired of crying."

There are so many levels to our losses; each requiring acceptance. Hanging onto and reliving those happy fun times over and over again is so inviting. We had such an easy and relaxed comfortable camaraderie that was laced with humor and laughter. As I move into the next season, it is so tempting to hang on to what was while recognizing the need to let go. It is time to let go. It is time to move forward.

Reflection and Personal Application

There have been many psychology and philosophy books written about the seasons of life. An untimely loss is a season thrust upon us that is out of sync with what we expect as a normal sequence of living. It is easier to accept losses that come with a natural progression of life. When aging takes a loved one, it is easier to accept and mourn that loss than when death is the result of a tragedy or other devastating set of circumstances.

Ecclesiastes writes about seasons that don't always fall within the normal expected course of life. We are reminded that no matter how we try to orchestrate our existence, it all ends in futility. But the author also lets us know that regardless of when a season occurs, there is something of importance we need to learn within each of them. We are encouraged not to hurry through them.

Life is about change and movement. Each season has a purpose. During those long winter months, we curl up in front of a cozy fireplace and read, study, or work on projects that out-of-door summer activities keep us from doing. In the spring, we are invigorated and ready to go outside. It is easier to prepare for seasons we expect. An out-of-sync season is an unimaginable intrusion in our otherwise defined expectation. Drastic and unwanted change is difficult to work through.

As we move from one season to another, we slowly and lovingly place all those wonderful things we treasured into our memories. Although it seems so final and conclusive, our losses are not diminished or forgotten. Instead we are building that transitional bridge from one period of time to another.

This new season offers the opportunity for deeper reflection of what life means to us personally and to discover more about ourselves. Start a new journal and put in it all the new discoveries you are making. Begin with the following list:

1. What new things are you learning about yourself that you were unaware of before?

2. What have you gained from your loss? What unexpected strengths are you discovering? Describe how you are still "okay" in spite of this transforming change.

3. What thoughts keep you bogged down in anxiety over what you should have done, wished you had done, or angry because you didn't do? Can you challenge them and offer yourself compassion as you let go?

4. What have you gained in resiliency, flexibility, tolerance, strength, faith, courage, and trust? As we grow and mature as a result of life's struggles, we tend to minimize these.

5. What have you learned about yourself that isn't so pleasing? It is time for acceptance of those things as well. Give yourself permission to be honest and offer yourself kindness and benevolence.

6. Can you find that kernel of humor each day, something that allows you to laugh? Put up jokes or humorous sayings around the house. Write them in your journal. Laugh at yourself when you make mistakes. Turn annoyance into humor whenever possible. Laughter washes away tension. It reduces obstacles and makes them more manageable. Humor empowers us to face our tomorrows regardless of what happens and enables us to turn our sorrow into something positive and healing.

CHAPTER 14

ENTWINING ROOTS

"For I will pour water on the thirsty ground and send streams
coursing through the parched earth. I will pour my Spirit into
your descendants and my blessing on your children. They shall
sprout like grass on the prairie, like willows alongside creeks."

ISAIAH 44:3–4 *THE MESSAGE*

There are two trees in my backyard. Their trunks touching, roots
entwining, they reach high into the sky, together yet separate. They
symbolize the life I shared with my husband. The love we shared was as
deep and connected as the entwining and supporting roots of these two
trees. We nurtured each other while allowing the other the independence
to grow in their own ways. One tree that was Le Roy has been cut down,
and the love that flowed through those roots that nourished each other
now seeps into barren soil.

A tree without water, Lord, slowly dies. You took the tree that stood
beside me, and there isn't another to replace it. And the lack of water, lack
of another intimate love, is slowly killing me. All the activities of the day
are just ways to stay alive in a world that demands movement or death
becomes inevitable.

Yet, I know that God is there beside me, even as I go on alone. I am amazed at how often I pick up a book and the words of encouragement I need to refresh and replenish my spirit are at my fingertips. New friends enter my life replacing old ones. I am given moments of respite and reflection that are healing balm to my battered spirit. I am supported as I struggle to put down new roots. They are not the entwining roots I shared with my husband, but new ones that will create a new support.

I remind myself that I am not alone and that every prayer I utter is a prayer received and answered in some way. It may not be the response I would like, but it is an answer that reflects positive changes that are constantly unfolding. My prayer now is that I recognize those positive changes.

Reflection and Personal Application

As the grief and loss journey proceeds over time, there will be moments when little things will acutely remind us of what we no longer have. But we also receive symbols of hope. On the day when I wrote this piece about entwining roots, it was the middle of winter. I had taken my little dog outside and the two trees in my back yard prompted a sharp reminder of what was no more. When I glanced at a nearby rose bush, I saw a solitary white rose blooming. While the trees were an indication of the relationship I shared with my husband, the rose became a symbol of hope for the future.

The love and acceptance my husband and I shared went beyond petty quarrels, cross words, or misunderstandings. Our relationship was more important than any momentary dispute or disagreements. There was a contentment just knowing the other was there. We held each other in high esteem and could share concerns and frustrations without criticism or callous judgment. We had a mutual respect for our individual professions and together established goals for our marriage and our family. When my husband died, I lost not only the man I loved but also my best friend.

When we lose someone we love, we lose a part of ourselves, our identity. That is true whether it is the death of a spouse, beloved sister, favored grandparent, wise parent, or best friend. Within such important liaisons we are free to be ourselves, warts and all.

Close relationships offer clarification, confidence, and encouragement. When there is respect, trust, and understanding, we can feel safe to share our hopes and dreams, doubts and fears as we explore aspirations or just share the trivialities of the day. It is where we learn about ourselves, our nice sides, and our not-so-nice sides. In the art of give-and-take, we discover the unexpected pleasure of giving for the sheer joy of giving. And in our squabbles, we learn how to negotiate and compromise. It takes time to build such enduring relations.

Grieving will become more challenging and arduous when we lose a marriage because of unfaithfulness or betrayal. We will feel dishonored and deceived, because a trust that was built has been betrayed. Such betrayals are devastating on many levels.

If the relationship you had with another had been rocky and troublesome, you might mourn the loss of what could have been. Divorces are endings between two people who were unable to develop a lasting connection that could endure through tough times as well as flourishing in good times. The inability to listen, respect differences, and get beyond diversities is often the cause for the death of a union that started with love and the best of intentions but ended in bitterness and hatred.

How do you grieve the loss of important relationships? How do you share with others what that bond had meant to you? Perhaps what is more important is that you define it for yourself. As you struggle through the many layers of loss, sorting through the good times and the bad times, you will be able to form a patchwork of life experiences that tell a story of what was shared.

In Chapter 8, I suggested ways to creatively express your feelings and commemorate your loss through some form of artistic endeavor such as a wall hanging or quilt or modeling clay. But there are other ways we can create a remembrance that can take the pieces of a life shared and place them lovingly into our memories, a visual way to bridge the gap from one chapter of our life story to another.

Here are some additional suggestions to enrich your memory bank

1. Start a scrap book and entitle it Memories or some other meaningful title. You might want to create a special box or other container that can hold pertinent information. You might include birth certificates, articles from the past, old letters, or anything that "captures" the spirit and essence of your loved one. This is for you; these are memories you want to keep that remind you of the person and the relationship you had.

2. You can do something similar to depict a life you once held that was important such as a marriage or a previous life of activity that is part of you but not viable today.

3. Write down some of the stories or bits and pieces you want to remember with fondness and appreciation. It might be some favorite sentences or words. Put these into your special remembrance book.

4. Start a memory book for your children or grandchildren that tell a visual story about their grandparent, aunt, uncle, or family friend who is deceased and who they will never have the opportunity to know. Share endearing parts of that life.

5. John James and Russell Friedman in their book, "The Grief Recovery Handbook", along with others speak to how writing a letter of goodbye to your loved one can be both healing and completing of a loss. Write a letter to your loved one. Tell him/her your thoughts and feelings. If your loss was the end of a marriage or the loss of your health, write to these. Put into your letter what this person, your marriage, or your health had meant to you. Allow yourself to be totally honest, because you are writing just for you. Imagine you are reading it to your loved one. In fact, it can be very therapeutic to read it out loud. The following are some things to consider as you write your letter.

- What I miss most about you is ...
- What I wish I'd said or hadn't said is ...
- What I remember most about our time together is ...
- What is hardest for me now is ...
- What I'd like to ask you is ...
- I'm keeping my memories of you alive by ...

Part III
From One Reality to Another—Redefining Ourselves

CHAPTER 15

SMOKE AND MIRRORS

"Smoke, nothing but smoke ... There's nothing to anything—it's
all smoke. What's there to show for a lifetime of work, a lifetime
of working your fingers to the bone? One generation goes its
way, the next one arrives, but nothing changes—
it's business as usual for old planet earth."

ECCLESIASTES 1:1–4 *THE MESSAGE*

Write? You want me to write, Lord? I'm not an accomplished writer,
and I haven't learned enough. What if I put down things that
expose my vulnerabilities, fears, ignorance, or just plain stupidity? With
all my education and learning, I have become acutely aware of just how
little I know. And just when I think I have learned a subject, I turn a page
and discover I have just begun.

The book of Ecclesiastes teaches us that striving after something is
like smoke and mirrors or dust blowing in the wind. Yet to survive in this
world, we are required to plan and work toward goals. We need to study
and learn and have a legitimate need to achieve and feel good about our
accomplishments.

But if we accumulate or accomplish simply for our own gratification
or the need to feel significant, we will wake up one morning disillusioned.

Ecclesiastes reveals that the meaning of life can only occur in, with, and through God.

As I pick up pen and paper, the boldness with which I have put down my thoughts and feelings in the past are now tempered with a deep humbling awareness of what I still need to learn.

I allow myself the freedom to express on paper what I have been experiencing throughout this journey, and I feel God guiding and helping me. I know that if I work in tandem with God, whatever I do will have meaning and purpose. Otherwise, my writing would only be tinsel and sparkle on paper that entertained for a moment but held nothing of value; and any accomplishments would be meaningless, dust blowing in the wind.

Journaling that began as therapy has now become a directive requiring the discipline of time, effort, and practice. As I shape and mold my stories, I am required to utilize the writing skills of proper sentence structure and good grammar, along with appropriate use of words. In the process, I am discovering more about myself.

And yet, is all this writing just smoke and mirrors? Is this really something I can aspire to? Or is it just an exciting interlude that will take me nowhere?

Reflection and Personal Application

Throughout recovery, we are moving from one sphere of existence to another. At first, we are simply trying to survive. Gradually, we progress beyond those lingering emotions of sadness, anger, shame, or guilt and shift toward finding a new way of life that will bring satisfaction.

Whenever one door closes, another opens. Leaving one world behind requires making the appropriate changes necessary to adapt to a new one. One of those changes is redefining who we are. We used to be a wife, husband, partner, good friend, parent, active and healthy person, etc. But who are we now? This is more than just life rearranging itself in a new way.

Our point of view, our perception of the world and possibilities for the future has all been altered. Some of the questions we face are: What is the same; what is different? What can I take with me from this tragedy that will make me a better person? Am I more compassionate and understanding of others? What have I discovered about myself that will enable me to make new meaningful goals for my future?

As we work through the complication of a new definition, we may place unrealistic expectations on ourselves or diminish our worth. It takes time to leave one established and satisfying lifestyle and move to another. This can be intimidating.

At first losses may seem like the end of the world with little promise for the future. It is easy to get discouraged while moving through this transition from old to new. Endless thoughts and questions bombard us. What is valid and what isn't? Is this worthwhile for me to pursue or is it just a passing fancy that holds no long-term fulfillment or satisfaction? Is there a way to test what is bone fide and real and what isn't? How do I confirm my abilities?

The following exercises can provide assistance:

1. Make a list of things you thought you might like to do some day. What interesting things have you dreamed of doing but never had the time or opportunity to do them? Perhaps you might explore them again. If you still have an interest, what would keep you from trying one on for size to see if it is as desirable as you once thought? There are many things we can do without investing a lot of finances. This is a time for exploration and experimentation. It is a time for testing what is important to you.

2. Continue to honor and respect your journey. As you experiment with new things, give yourself permission to fail. Don't be judgmental of any initial efforts. Avoid critical self-talk such as: *I'm so stupid, I screwed up again, I never do anything right, or why did I think I could do this.*

3. Write a letter to yourself describing how you feel today and how you felt yesterday. Remind yourself of all your assets and the growth you've made. Put in this letter all the reasons you are

proud of who you are and what you are accomplishing. It takes courage to try new things. Give yourself a mental pat on the back for the things you are willing to try each day, no matter how trivial it may seem. You are building on the strengths you already have and not allowing setbacks to change the core of who you are. Ask God to strengthen your resolve.

4. Find new ways to nurture your spirit. Create hope and faith statements, such as: *God loves me, I expect good things to happen, I am not alone,* and *these difficult times will pass.* Repeat them often during the day. Copy favorite verses from a book or Scripture and post them around the house. Remember, it takes a lot of little steps to get to a destination. We do not need to run a marathon.

CHAPTER 16

PATH? WHAT PATH?

"And don't for a minute let this Book of Revelation be out of
mind. Ponder and meditate on it day and night, making sure
you practice everything written in it. Then you'll get where
you're going; then you'll succeed. Haven't I commanded you?
Strength! Courage! Don't be timid; don't get discouraged. GOD
your God, is with you every step you take."

JOSHUA 1:8–9 *THE MESSAGE*

Before we take any trip, we have a destination in mind; we know where
we are going. We have considered the best route and what we need
to take with us. With a schedule in hand, we know when we are going to
leave and return. Then, we make reservations and pack our bags.

The trip of life, however, isn't quite so easy or direct. Often, it seems
as though we are wandering in a no-man's land that stretches into infinity,
devoid of markers or signposts. We take the first path we see, not sure
where we want to go or where we will end up, but hoping it will take us to
a life that is fulfilling and satisfying. Too often, however, we find ourselves
at a dead end needing to start over again.

God chose Joshua to lead the people of Israel out of the desert where
they had been wandering for forty years and into the Promised Land.

But as they stood at the banks of the roaring Jordan River, swollen with early spring rains, and looked across to the other side, it wasn't a land of milk and honey they saw, but a land of giants, walled cities, undefeated kings and well-trained armies. In short, insurmountable odds. Was this the pathway to their new life? I'm sure Joshua, for all his bravery, might have asked, "God, is this really where you want us to go?"

As a new writer, I am entering a land of giants, a world of talented and gifted people who seem to have it all together; while I, on the other hand, struggle with putting down on paper my thoughts and ideas. The pathway seems like sand and rocks and raging rivers, the obstacles of publication as large as any giant army or walled city without markers. This land of writing is already inhabited by men and women successful in their trade. They are the giants with whom I would have to compete. And like Joshua, I ask, "God is this really where you want me to go?

But God sees far beyond the horizon. He knows the path we are to take even when we can't see it. He gives us glimpses of possibilities of what our lives could be if we trusted and stepped out in faith. But the choice is ours: we can continue to wander around in our own deserts or cross over into new terrain.

Reflection and Personal Application

I had been a college teacher, a licensed counselor and facilitator of many groups. Now I felt I was being called to enter a new way of life. Serious writing as an author was intimidating. It was walking away from the safety and security of what I knew and crossing the River Jordan into a new existence.

Endings can be scary. We want to return to what we knew and what was comfortable. But the past as we knew it no longer exists. There is no going back. The world in which we had moved is not the same.

Each stage of life, from infancy through adulthood, has certain tasks to be accomplished so we can adjust to the next level of growth and development. With each step, we take what we have learned and apply it in some way. In the process, we develop frames of reference that direct our behaviors in response to our encounters with life. As a deeper appreciation and interpretation is gained of who we are and who we can become our frames of reference expand. These are often referred to as "turning points" or "defining moments."

"Frame of reference" is a term used to describe how we identify and evaluate incoming information. What do we let in and what do we exclude? This not only helps to regulate our behavior, but it also enables us to anticipate and react appropriately to circumstances and establish the rules to live by. Our frames of reference can be narrow and rigid or open and expansive.

All the experiences, emotions, and information that we have collected over the years is stored and organized in our brain. As we grow up, core beliefs are established about how we fit into the world and our sense of self-worth and personal control. The events and people who have interacted with us since infancy help influence, shape and fashion us into the individuals we are today.

Loss interjects itself into this normal progression and demands the need for a new interpretation. Like the Israelites crossing the river Jordon who saw giants and armies and walled cities, we look at the changes required of us and feel vulnerable, intimated, anxious, and afraid. It is not only life that has been changed dramatically with this loss, but also me. And yet, this very loss gives us an opportunity to see a broader picture, change directions or choose different options to apply ourselves in more meaningful ways.

So, ask yourself these questions: What new frame of reference is required by your loss? What expectations and assumptions we had no longer exist? Who am I today without that beloved person beside me? How has that accident or debilitating disease changed how I view myself? As we struggle to adjust and accommodate our thinking for this new reality, we are adjusting not just to a new world but a new defining identity.

As we enter a transitional phase, our focus shifts from the past to the here and now and a new outlook. In this timeframe, our tasks require reflection and redefining our identities, roles, and significant values. Our frames of reference will be enlarged. It is a time to be alone, but not necessarily lonely. The time spent here may seem unproductive but is so important to help bridge the gap between the past and the present, between our old life and a new life.

It is estimated that major life transitions take from eighteen months to four years to complete. We get impatient and want to move on in a couple of weeks or months. But each journey requires its own time frame, and we can only benefit when we grant ourselves the time we need.

You may be called to walk on a new path, to expand your horizon and try new things. Here are some things to consider as you contemplate and reflect:

1. What part of the past is keeping you stuck and preventing you from moving forward?

2. What fears are keeping you from crossing the bridge to a new life?

3. What old beliefs, lifestyles, life scripts, assumptions, expectations, etc. are prohibiting you from exploring new options? Life scripts tell us what we should do, have to do or must do. Life scripts can be rewritten.

4. Who do you want to become? Give yourself permission to explore.

5. What new path and opportunities can you envision? Start making a list and expand it every day. We choose to remain stuck or move forward.

CHAPTER 17

SEAGULLS ON THE WIND

"As for man, his days are like grass; he flourishes like a flower of
the field; for the wind passes over it, and it is gone, and its place
knows it no more. But the steadfast love of the LORD is from
everlasting to everlasting upon those who fear him."

PSALM 103:15–17

This morning, my thoughts and feelings ebb and flow like the tides of
the ocean. I close my eyes and allow pictures from the past to enter
my consciousness. I see seagulls wheeling and soaring above the ocean
waves. On the sandy beaches below patterns and ridges are shaped by
incoming tides. At the ocean's edge, sea grasses dance in the wind, weaving shadows of beauty and grace on the endless sand. The sun kisses the
tips of the waves turning them into sparkling diamonds.

As my view expands, I see inland an eagle soaring high above a river,
its eyes focused on the ripples of water and the signs of fish swimming
upstream. In one determined and skillfully executed dive, he retrieves a
salmon for his dinner.

In my imagination, I let go and become one of those seagulls carried
by the wind over cresting waves, soaring high above the earth. I experience a sense of freedom and lightness as I soar above and over my losses

and sadness. I look down and see God's love sprinkled everywhere over his creation. It leaves a residue on the sands of my soul just as the surf leaves a residue of foam and seaweed on the shoreline. That love reminds me that God is as faithful as the tides. This residue becomes the memory that sustains me when the night is at its blackest and the storms crash over me with such intensity I think I shall never survive.

It is said that God carries us during tough times, and he certainly has carried me. Just as the love I had experienced with my loved one remains as memories etched forever in my heart, the love God displays through-out his creation continue to create memories of hope that draw me out from under the crashing waves of distress to soar high above.

Lord, help me to remember, that I do not have to remain in the crashing waves but can rise above any troubles. I can soar above the things that anchor me to anxiety and uncertainty. I can soar into the heavens and feel your love give me freedom to ascend above whatever I am experiencing at the moment. I can let go and fly.

Reflection and Personal Application

In those early days of loss, we may feel as though we have been flung on the beaches of life by crashing and destructive waves. All we see is our well thought out plans and goals hurled on the sands like so much debris. But if, after the winds and water have calmed, we could soar above our tragedy, we would have an expanded view revealing a well-ordered world that includes both storms and calm seas; we would see more than just the wreckage left by the storm.

We want neat tidy endings, and transitions that move us along in a predictable fashion. But reclaiming our life is not a step-by-step process that takes us from one place to another in an orderly, sequential fashion. It is going in and out, examining past experiences and knowledge gained, so we can forge them together into a new beginning. By joining together the old and new, the life lived and the life yet to live, we become the best of both.

Making that transition from what we loved and cherished to an unknown future can be daunting and intimidating. Sometimes in our haste to get away from what was destroyed by adversity, we miss the insight, understanding, and wisdom we are gaining.

As we pick up the pieces of our life, we may find some pieces no longer relevant or important. We can choose those that expand who we are, that clarify our values and give us a more compassionate understanding of our existence.

Visualization can be very helpful in this process. When we create positive pictures in our minds, we are physically and mentally drawn towards those images.

Here are some ways to create positive pictures to move toward:

1. Using the relaxation techniques given in Chapter Four, close your eyes and allow your mind and body to relax. Visualize yourself walking along the beach. What items do you see strewn around? Which ones could be made into a new piece of art? Pick up the pieces you are drawn to and see yourself creating an attractive piece of sculpture, arrangement, or picture from them. It may require some carving, sanding, additional molding and polishing. What was broken has become an exquisite new piece of art. Step back and enjoy what you have created.

   Now, imagine that this new creation is you. You are that magnificent treasure, newly sculpted and re-arranged. What pieces were irrelevant, no longer needed and were left behind? What was tenderly reworked with great care and love? What was added to enhance and make you more defined and exquisite? See yourself as this newly fashioned work of art, woven into a beautiful rich tapestry of old and new.

   Hang this beautiful new portrait of you filled with hope, wisdom and high regard, on the wall of your mind. Then open your eyes and return to the present moment.

2. Reflect on all the ways you can accomplish future goals. In

your personal journal, write down the core values, beliefs, and principles you want to bring to this life. Create a mission statement for yourself that outlines how you will live those principles.

3. Focus on what you can do instead of what you can't do. Make a purposeful commitment to eliminate the word *can't* from your vocabulary. Replace with "*I can.*" Can't is a stone wall—we can soar over stone walls, go around or eliminate them. Making a decision about things we don't want to do is different than saying we can't do something.

4. Return to your "new you" visualization as often as possible; but especially when you feel overwhelmed about thoughts of the future. Remind yourself you have not been destroyed but renewed. See yourself doing and living with a new purpose. Imagine how you feel as you walk toward a brighter future.

CHAPTER 18

IN THE STORM OF LIFE

"GOD addressed Job from the eye of the storm."

JOB 40:6, *THE MESSAGE*

It is within the eye of the hurricane where the promise of peace lies for a brief moment, a respite before the next onslaught of the storm.

I have been struck by hurricane force winds that took my husband and now threaten to destroy the remainder of my life. The fury of those swirling currents picked up my dreams and smashed them like matchsticks.

Then the winds calmed, and I was lulled into thinking the worst had past and I was safe from its battering assault. But I was only in the eye of the storm. Within its calm, I was given a new friend. Together we supported one another as we shared our stories of faith, hope, pain, and lost dreams. It was a time of reprieve and deceptive peace.

The eye passed, and once again I was thrown into the destructive force of turbulent events that uprooted even more of my world. Cancer invaded my daughter's life. The fervor of the winds shook our faith and threatened to unsettle our trust in God.

But the God who was there in the beginning of the tempest, and stayed with me in the lull, now guided my daughter through surgery, chemotherapy, radiation, and healing. He helped me with the sale of my home and the construction of a new one. God never left us. And as the winds finally ceased, I was set down, safe and intact, with a new hip, a new home, and a calmness to survey my new world; a new beginning.

As I pause to survey the new space where I find myself, I am thankful the hurricane has passed. I feel the sun shining on the remnants of my former life. Even when a cloud covers the sun and threatens to steal my hope for a future, I am reminded that storms come and go. And when the winds of life rise again, I will remember there is always a new day to start over.

Reflection and Personal Application

Storms are part of our lives. We can liken them to tornadoes, hurricanes, or seas whipped into overpowering waves. While each of us may describe our storms differently, the result is the same; our life suffers devastation of some kind. Even when we know we will experience such storms, we are often unprepared for their severity and how quickly in succession they can occur.

In working with people over the years, I have observed how often several catastrophes occur within a short period of time. When tragedies create a snowball effect, there is little time to pull ourselves together before experiencing another onslaught. You have just begun to pick up the pieces before being hit again.

It isn't just new disasters that impact grieving a major loss, but old, unresolved wounds and injuries from our childhood that resurface. These can be as simple as the loss of a favorite pet never reconciled as a child to a death of a family member or the divorce of parents.

Old Losses

Children do not have the maturity to separate themselves from events and will often attribute bad things that happen as being their fault. This is especially true when parents divorce – children attribute it to being their fault. These old sources of doubts and shame can be felt again.

Children have difficulty expressing what they are experiencing, and parents, in their desire to shield them from painful feelings, often try to protect them by making light of difficult situations or excluding them from discussions. Consoling statements made do not allow the child to express what they may be feeling about what was lost.

"We can get you another dog (pet)," or "Here is a cookie. Don't cry, everything is going to be okay," or "Grandma just fell asleep." These statements can be confusing to a child who is hurt, upset, scared, and trying to understand what has happened. Because they have difficulty putting feelings into words, children act out what they are feeling or withdraw and become further isolated in misunderstanding. Unresolved, painful events become buried, and when we experience losses as adults, these old incidents are often triggered again demanding attention.

What messages about grieving did you hear when you were growing up? What did you observe through actions or words of those around you that indicated you were not to feel, cry, or otherwise express sorrow over what was taken away? How did family and friends handle grief? Did their denial or lack of conversation help them recover or did it keep their feelings locked up? Exploring these old ways of dealing with grief can give you insight into how you may want to deal with yours.

Childhood Abuse

Childhood traumas of physical, sexual, verbal, or emotional abuse are often hidden, buried beneath feelings of shame and unworthiness. They were unspoken of as though silence may somehow make them not real. Because incidents of abuse remain unacknowledged, the feelings triggered can be confusing and difficult. We thought they were in the past. We didn't want to deal with them. When such events from our past are triggered, it complicates our grief and we can become traumatized all over again.

At first, the emotions from past traumas will flood our consciousness before we remember the details of such events. Within such traumas are conflicting thoughts and unresolved questions along with confusing emotions of anger, shame, rejection, guilt, rage, hatred, and inappropriate love.

If you feel such emotional memories from past traumas are surfacing, please seek the assistance of a professionally trained therapist to help work through such events. Working through them will give you the freedom at last to heal and explore the wonderful unique person you are.

Cumulative Effects of Losses

It is hard to remain hopeful when hit with many losses on many different fronts. It is easy to become bitter and cynical; life is unfair and why me. But cynicism, if we allow it residence, only increases our pain and creates doubt, distrust, and pessimism about any future happiness. Bitterness and resentment build giant barriers in making a new beginning. We can counteract this by purposefully looking for the positive in whatever is happening.

In Chapter three, I suggested starting a gratitude journal. If you haven't already done so, I would encourage you to begin. Seeking and revealing the good that is there within the hurt promotes a healthy attitude and wellbeing. Research shows that consciously seeking and focusing on the blessings in our life and developing the skill of gratitude are enormously beneficial not only to our state of mind, but our physical health as well.

Shifting your focus to things you can be thankful for is not constructing a Pollyanna outlook with unrealistic optimism. Instead, it is establishing a mindset and attitude that brings faith, trust and hope to our efforts and our future. When pessimistic negative thoughts are replaced with realistic expectations our self-talk will change from thoughts of "what will I do or what will happen to me" to "I can make it. I will survive. I will be happy again." It restores energy and possibility. Ongoing negative thinking suppresses anticipation and optimism and fuels hopelessness, helplessness and depression.

Here are some things to consider:

1. Add to your gratitude journal not only blessings in the moment, but also constructive and supportive memories from the past. Reflect on those times when you enjoyed happiness and joy with your loved ones. Affirm your ability to experience laughter,

humor and happiness in the future. Continue to look for ways each day to find things to laugh about. As mentioned before, laughter is emotionally, spiritually, and physically healing.

2. Make a conscious and deliberate choice to let go of bitterness, unfairness and injustice. Hanging onto grievances, no matter how justified, will eventually destroy you. One of our greatest attributes is to choose new responses. While it may be difficult to come to terms with senseless acts of violence, major natural disasters, or simply ongoing bad personal disasters, you can choose not to let it rule your life. Let go. Forgiveness is for you and is necessary to enjoy life again.

3. Repeating affirmations often during the day can bring a different perspective or assessment of what is happening. They can draw us toward a different and more productive and positive outcome. Use the examples below or write your own. Write affirmations in first person, "I", and write them as if they were already true. It may make you feel uncomfortable at first because you don't feel that way as yet, but remember affirmations draw you toward that state of mind and presence that will move you in the direction you want to go.

Here are some basic examples to begin your list:

- I give myself time to grieve and heal
- I am feeling better every day
- I find things to be grateful for every day
- I find the help I need
- I have many abilities. I weigh options and make good decisions
- Continue to create new affirmations as you go along that are pertinent to where you are and what you are doing. This is an ongoing process.

CHAPTER 19

THERAPY OF WRITING

"For Isaiah, words are watercolors and melodies and chisels to
make truth and beauty and goodness. He creates visions,
delivers revelation, arouses belief. He is a poet."

EUGENE PETERSON, "INTRODUCTION TO ISAIAH," *THE MESSAGE*

W riting every morning has become a ritual. I feel incomplete without it. It is both a solace and a new beginning. It stabilizes me
while I sweep away the lint and dust balls of depressive thinking that col-
lect and hide in the corners of my brain. It is a time of transformation:
finding "me", discovering my imagination and resourcefulness as I learn
more about God.

Writing takes the filing cabinets of my mind and empties the drawers
filled with junk that clutter thinking and restricts perspective and clarity.
Jumbled thoughts continue to jostle for attention: reflections on my life
together with my husband, what I want to do in the future, and exploring
options. As I shuffle through the bits and pieces of my life, I give myself
permission to keep what I need and want while letting go of the frivolous.
Feelings of tranquility and positive expectations fill my mind and spirit.

What started as simple therapy through journaling has now become
a requirement; an ongoing productive exercise. Journaling allowed

thoughts to flow in incoherent ways. Purposeful writing takes scattered memories and life experiences and transforms them into a cohesive narrative. It expands my field of vision to see beyond telephoto snapshots of loss to a panoramic view of God's overall plan for us of which I am a part.

My pen is the brush I use to boldly paint on new canvas being woven. As developing stories take shape, my losses become a defining feature. Exploring new possibilities through writing melds together the past and present and forms a cohesiveness and appreciation of what I have that I can use as I create my new reality.

Reflection and Personal Application

Spring is the sign of a new beginning – rebirth – a time when what seemed dead produces new growth. It is a time of pruning old growth, moving aside dead leaves and tending new shoots. We give a boost of plant food to stimulate that new growth.

Expanding our writing is like brushing away the dead debris accumulated from the winter so that we can discover new dimensions of ourselves. The following exercise can begin a new journey into spring.

First thing in the morning before you do anything else, take paper and pencil and start writing whatever comes to your mind, whether it makes sense of not. You may find yourself beginning with words such as, "This is a stupid exercise, but here I am ..."

First introduced by Julia Cameron in her book, *The Artist's Way*, it is an exercise I have used for myself and given to clients and students. Write with no restrictions and no pre-determination until you fill three pages. It is a powerful exercise that allows great insight while releasing creativity and understanding.

This exercise may uncover old habits from your past that are impeding your progress. Old ways of looking at ourselves, replaying of negative tapes from our past, self-debasing self-talk rehearsed and repeated over and over again. You may become conscious of fixed and rigid beliefs that contain labels given to us in school or at home that tell us we are dumb or stupid. We continue to believe them because we have rehearsed them so often. Every time we repeat them, we remind ourselves about all the times we have failed and how incompetent we are. As these messages become more dominant over time, they formulate predictions of what we can and cannot do in the future.

Here are some ways to challenge old patterns of destructive thinking. For example, to challenge thinking that says you are stupid and always screw up, ask yourself, where did these thoughts come from? Who says you are stupid? Was this something you were repeatedly told as a child? How accurate and truthful are they? Then replace negative thoughts with more logical and realistic ones, such as the ones below:

- *While I did dumb things as a kid, that was when I was a kid.*
- *I have made and continue to make good choices.*
- *I have learned a lot over the years and am quite capable of making good choices.*
- *When I make a mistake, I am able to learn something valuable from it.*
- *I am learning to appreciate who I am and make choices that are right for me.*

When our thinking and the beliefs that drive them are products of our past, we can get stuck in an ongoing cycle. When we challenge them, we are examining and looking at them from today's standpoint. We can then replace with correcting information and change both negative beliefs and thought patterns. Forgiveness, unexpected blessings, gratitude, temperance, flexibility, and grace become part of that new narrative and perspective.

It is easy to find fault with ourselves and others when looking backward. Recovery is balancing our perceptions of self-recriminations or blame with reasonable objectivity. Unless we challenge pervasive negative thoughts, they will remain habits that continue to corrode our lives.

Continuing to focus on doubts and thoughts about what we should or shouldn't have done before our loss or when our loved one was sick is normal and natural. However, if we don't resolve them and they continue to dominate our thinking over a long period of time without resolution, we again become a victim to them. The following are some examples of such thoughts people may experience during grief.

- *I didn't do enough.*
- *I wish I had done ...*
- *I don't know what to do now.*
- *I don't want things to change.*
- *How will I face the rest of my life?*
- *I will never experience laughter or be happy again.*
- *I will never experience joy or love again.*

The examples below illustrate how we can challenge and replace those and other negative thoughts with more realistic and positive ones.

- *I didn't do enough.* I did everything I could, given my circumstances, what I knew, and was capable of doing at the time.
- *I wish I had done ...* It is always easier to look backward and believe I could have done more or done things differently. I did all I could at the time.
- *I don't know what to do now.* I know it will be tough, but I have tackled difficult things in the past. I can ask opinions of my friends, get advice from reputable sources, and begin to evaluate different options.
- *I don't want things to change.* Nobody wants good things to come to an end, but without change I will not have the opportunity to expand who I am. I wouldn't be able to experience something new. There is good in this ending. The future can be positive again.

- *How will I face the rest of my life?* I have loyal friends and will meet new friends. With support, I can face anything.
- *Will I ever be happy again? So much of what was meaningful to me was tied up in my loss.* I have had losses in the past and have created new beginnings that were not only meaningful but also satisfying. I can do it again.
- *Will I ever feel love and joy again?* I am still the same person capable of love. Right now, I will focus on loving myself, meeting my needs, and taking care of myself. I will allow others to help me, and I will reach out to others. I will experience happiness, satisfaction, and contentment again.

Consider the following:

1. What thoughts about my loss keep recurring over and over again? How accurate or true are they? Are they slanted or biased against me or others?
2. What destructive emotions am I experiencing because of habitual negative thinking? Take one of them, challenge its validity, and replace it with a more positive thought. Then take another and do the same.
3. What new action can I take right now to think positively about my future? What will I see happening?
4. Keep a log of emotions that continue to be pervasive and disruptive. When are they triggered? What thoughts are associated with them? Challenge and replace the negative thoughts with constructive ones. For example, "I am so angry that the accident happened that took the life of my loved one." Reframe and replace with, "I am angry, but it is time to use this as a positive force to help and support others." Expanding your frame of reference is taking it out of the "telephoto" lens of your life camera and putting it into "wide angle" so you can see more of the picture.

CHAPTER 20

MY SPECIAL PLACE

"Oh, visit the earth; ask her to join the dance! Deck her out in
spring showers; fill the God-River with living water. Paint the
wheat fields golden. Creation was made for this! Drench the
plowed fields; soak the dirt clods with rainfall as harrow and
rake bring her to blossom and fruit. Snow-crown the peaks with
splendor, scatter rose petals down your paths, all though the
wild meadows, set the hills to dancing."

PSALM 65:9–12 THE MESSAGE

The sun is streaming through my window this morning. It is still cold
outdoors, but my fireplace warms my heart as it heats my bedroom.
Patterns of light and shadow form on the walls, creating pieces of moving
art as the wind rustles the trees outside. I snuggle deeper into my chair
with my comforter and steaming cup of coffee and watch in fascination as
pine needles and branches form dancing silhouettes above my bed.

The heavy cloud cover in the Northwest can make the winter months
gray and dark. But when the sun breaks through, everything that had
been dreary and dull comes alive. The threads in my comforter shine like
gold, and my home is colored with richness as the sun's rays penetrate
deep into every room.

In the same way, my life becomes highlighted with new brilliance and texture when God's rays reach through the curtains of gloom to dance on the walls of my heart. How hard it is to define such a love that can make things come alive! When besieged with monumental losses or endless problems, our world may seem cold and pale. At such times, I need to remind myself that just as the physical sun continues to shine above the grey clouds, God's love continues to shine on me when the days seem the darkest and longest. I can choose how I respond to those dark clouds and turn even long winter days into blessings.

Reflection and Personal Application

In making my transition from loss to a new beginning, I didn't just want to recover from grief - I wanted to live again. The days can seem long and progress questioned as we go through the transitional period. Reflecting on past accomplishments reminded me of other times when I faced adversity and not only survived but thrived. When strengths used in the past are remembered, it can be a source of encouragement in the present.

Loss creates doubts in our competence and abilities. While it is normal and natural to doubt, we can allow them to throw a deep cloud of reservation over what we believe we can and cannot do.

No matter how bad things may seem in the present, there were many times in the past when you not only overcame but prospered. You made goals and met them. You have many strengths and attributes. They are waiting to be put to use again.

The following exercises can help identify past accomplishments and help you affirm the skills and talents you already possess.

1. Make a list of all your past accomplishments. Reflect on the risks involved, the struggles, and the challenges associated with them. These are not trivial or small accomplishments; they are important. It is time to think about them as successes.
2. Make a list of all your strengths, both personal and professional.

Don't minimize any of them. Losses can diminish our evaluation of what we are capable. Celebrate all of you.

3. Focus your thoughts on future possibilities. You might feel at times as though you are barely surviving, but that will change as energy and motivation return.

4. Ask good friends to make a list of the attributes they admire in you. Reflect on these as validation of your worth as seen from another's eyes affirming how much you are appreciated and valued by others. You are necessary. You are needed.

Part IV
A New Beginning

CHAPTER 21

SURROUNDED BY BLESSINGS

"God, my God, how great you are! Beautifully, gloriously robed,
dressed up in sunshine, and all heaven stretched out for your
tent. You built your palace on the ocean deeps, made a chariot
out of clouds and took off on wind-wings. You commandeered
winds as messengers, appointed fire and flame as ambassadors.
What a wildly wonderful world, God! You made it all,
with Wisdom at your side."

PSALM 104:1–4, 24 *THE MESSAGE*

It's raining. The gentle patter of raindrops refreshes my soul as it does the humid summer air. I listen to soothing sounds through my open window. The mayhem of rushing people and activities is tuned out, and I focus on the peaceful sounds that surround me.

Every day we are witness to many blessings that fall like gentle drops of rain or silently tumbling snowflakes. Who hasn't felt refreshed after a summer rain shower or been touched by the quiet serenity of an earth blanketed in mounds of downy snow that shimmers like diamonds in the winter sun? Who hasn't experienced the deep, enduring, and gentle peace that comes from looking over a countryside bathed in the light of a full moon? And what person hasn't marveled at stars so dazzling and vivid it seems we could reach up and touch them. At such times, nature is silenced and time suspended.

Yet, the snow is only frozen water, and the sun, moon, and stars are nothing more than hardened, desolate, uninhabitable rocks and dangerous gasses. What transforms these unattractive objects into things of beauty? What happens to change the mundane of everyday events into things of beauty, miracles and blessings?

When I allow my mind to become attuned to what is happening around me, I find myself in tune with God and am rewarded with a profound connection and healing of mind and spirit. And I am comforted through the timeless tranquility and harmony of creation. As God reveals himself through such eternal and enduring acts every day, we are witness to the mystery of life constantly unfolding around us—from the green shoot pushing up through the dirt to the developing baby spiders clinging precariously to the edge of their webs.

Reflection and Personal Application

When loss is fresh, the world seems stark and barren and we struggle to see anything of beauty or value. Instead of sparkling snow and twinkling stars, we feel bitter cold and endless dark skies. The summer rain is an intrusion on activities; the baby spiders are nuisances to be quickly swept away; and the garden only sprouts weeds.

What transforms the ordinary and commonplace into special events? One moment my spirit is dejected and feeling despair, the next I am feeling calm and serene. What changes those responses?

Perhaps it is when we recognize that our loss isn't the end of the world; that the events can be turned into something different by how we look at it. In the middle of a storm, I just want to survive. When the assault ends, at first I only see destruction. But as I work with the remains, I begin to see more: new growth, new opportunity, new depth of living and experiencing.

Blessings are in the midst of us all the time if we choose to be a witness.

Making it a habit requires continuing the practice for the rest of our lives. It isn't just an exercise while going through tough times. Recognizing blessings and expressing gratitude becomes a lifestyle.

Life as usual will continue with storms and cold winter nights that give us pause to mourn, evaluate and grow. But we can take the valuable lessons we have learned and apply them on an on-going basis. Patience, looking beyond the moment, staying calm, and working on solutions can be great assets. We can apply the strength, compassion and expanded point of view to everyday living with friends and family and anyone else we meet.

The lessons we have learned have value. In extending compassion towards yourself you can now extend that same compassion and understanding to others. As we have learned to be comforted, we can comfort those who need comforting. The extended frame of reference, new mindsets and attitudes we have gained for ourselves can now help others who are struggling with self-esteem and worth.

We can listen with respect and attention instead of becoming defensive or judgmental. We can let go of the negative and focus on the underneath issues of pain someone may be experiencing. We can become sensitive to others who are struggling with losses and be a supportive friend. I can extend grace as I have extended grace to myself. I can purposefully look for the good in others instead of focusing only on what is wrong. And I can seek those things that remain constant and never changing instead of concentrating on disorder and confusion.

Good things do come out of disasters and misfortunes. Like the snow, we can see sparkling diamonds of opportunity or just bitter cold and black skies. We can see God working for good in our lives like tiny new green spring sprouts instead of misfortunes. We can create anticipation and optimism instead of looking only at the bittersweet. We can make our lives into frozen, uninhabitable landscapes or turn them into living pictures of inspiration, hopefulness, and positive expectation. And we can lift others up as we have been lifted up.

Some things to consider as we reconstruct our lives:

1. Make a list of ways you can take your new understanding, attitudes, and viewpoints and use them in developing better relationships.

2. How can you change your conversations and interactions to make them more positive, both for yourself and for the other?

3. Celebrate your loss. Celebrations are not just marking a special day on the calendar. It is finding a way to show happiness over what you had. It doesn't have to be noisy or boisterous. Here are some ways to celebrate:

4. Host a dinner party. On the anniversary of the death of my husband, I invited all our boating friends over for a dinner. We toasted as we laughed about the funny boating experiences we had shared, even those that weren't so funny. We laughed and cried and loved him all over again.

5. With the premature loss of a baby, celebrate your baby's life by creating a baby book of thoughts and wishes and dreams and pictures of what might have been. Write your baby a letter and say how much you loved him or her. Plant a shrub, a rose bush, or a tree or place a piece of art in a favored spot as a remembrance and smile as you go by.

6. If you have gone through a divorce, spend time reflecting on everything that went *right*. Remember all the love and good expectations you brought to that marriage. You still have them. You can take them with you into any new relationship.

7. If a chronic illness or loss of limb has taken away your ability to function, remember you are not reduced in the process. Focus on those things you are able to do, no matter how trivial or small they may seem. Celebrate each one. Celebrate you. Celebrate others.

CHAPTER 22

ON TOP OF THE MOUNTAIN

"Moses climbed from the Plains of Moab to Mount Nebo,
the peak of Pisgah facing Jericho. GOD
showed him all the land."

DEUTERONOMY 34:1 *THE MESSAGE*

L earning new skills requires determination, struggle, and hard work. It seems at times that we push and push that proverbial stone and it doesn't move. And then, one morning, we wake up and find ourselves sitting on top of it! We haven't moved it; we haven't gone around it; we have climbed on top and are on our way over and beyond.

That's how I feel this morning. I have reached the top! I don't know how I got here, but here I am. Every morning I have written about my struggle to believe, make sense of what happened, let go, and move forward. It was a new skill I was perfecting as I grieved my loss.

I sit on top of this mountain, my proverbial rock, and look back and see the black canyons, deep abysses, and steep trails that have challenged me. I see what I couldn't see while climbing those often treacherous paths: the guardrails God put up for my protection, the "angels" he sent to comfort me, and the green pastures that were sweet resting places along the way. He put people in my life for assistance and support to just "be there" for me. He provided protection, love, and strength to endure.

During this grieving time, I have asked myself challenging questions. My mental, emotional, and physical resources were stretched to the max, and at the end of the day I would fall into bed exhausted only to wake in the morning and start all over again. At times the trail seemed endless or too steep, and I would ask myself, *how will I make it through another day*? But standing still was never an option and with steel determination I moved forward.

Looking back at my journey, I remember there had been patches of blue sky. When I had looked up instead of down, confusing and bewildering pathways were clarified, and I was able to move through my pain and learn from it. My faith and trust were sharpened when traveling confusing and bewildering pathways; and I was given new energy and hope when I had to climb over obstacles of doubt and uncertainty. And when the trail seemed to disappear from sight, God gave toeholds and branches to grab hold of and hang on to until the path was made clear again.

I shake off the residue of sadness. I want to run like the spring colts I see galloping across the fields near my home. I can see myself racing with them, high spirited and exuberant, full of excitement for no reason other than being alive.

Reflection and Personal Application

The time comes when we realize winter has past and spring has arrived. The snow has melted and crocuses and daffodils poke their heads out of the cold ground. Budding trees seem ready to explode with new color. The last winds of winter have lost their bite and warm air prevails.

Our lives, too, experience a renewal. The harshness of grief has melted and is replaced with the warm winds of hope and optimism. Emerging from winter's clutches, we see an expansive panoramic view of what we can become. Loss may give us short pause in the scheme of things; but it allows us to consider and examine what a meaningful life means. We are taking charge of our lives and hold a new appreciation and understanding of what we have gone through and what we have gained from it.

As you view all the options available to you, consider the following:

1. Write a personal mission statement, declaring your refusal to be a victim and your desire to live to the fullest. This is a formal declaration that you date and sign. Tell yourself you want to make the changes that will improve your ongoing life and make you happy.

2. Re-examine those hidden dreams once more you may have denied up till now because you thought they were too outrageous or frivolous. Can you now allow yourself to make them happen? Remember President George W. Bush made his first skydive at the age of 80. Age is not a barrier unless we make it. Finances can be budgeted to include what is truly important to us.

3. What are the goals you want to make? The time has come to explore and take great leaps of faith. Don't prejudge. Anything is possible if you can dream and visualize it.

4. We are made whole when we give back to others. Perhaps this is a time to put into action those thoughts about starting a charity or joining a movement that can bring about positive change for the poor, homeless or down and out. Take that new energy and use it to accomplish amazing things, not just for yourself, but for others.

CHAPTER 23

A FRESH START

"Oh! Teach us to live well! Teach us to live wisely and well!
Come back, GOD—how long do we have to wait? ... Surprise us
with love at daybreak; then we'll skip and dance all the day long.
Make up for the bad times with some good times; we've seen
enough evil to last a lifetime. Let your servants see what you're
best at, the ways you rule and bless your children."

PSALM 90:12–16 THE MESSAGE

The sun is shining. I have swept the cobwebs from my mind, and I stand within clean rooms. I have examined my past and retain those things that are important to me; labeled and filed for easy access and reference should I need them. Rules, unrealistic expectations, and life scripts that no longer apply have been thrown out. I open the windows of my soul and allow the fresh air of new beginnings to stream in.

Although the future remains uncertain, I meet it with a new attitude and mindset. I have replaced old beliefs and assumptions with more realistic and practical ones. New dreams have been substituted for those that have outlived their time. Fears and anxieties that no longer serve a purpose dissipate into the mists of time.

I am not alone in my new beginning, for God continues to walk beside me. His grace and wisdom illuminate the route I take. His love pours through the chinks and cracks of my heart, permeating every cell of my body and filling my spirit with hope.

When the cold winds of another icy winter bring future heartbreaks and disappointments, the memory of this sun will continue to burn warm and bright. It will guide and sustain me as I remember that winters do pass, and new springs do arrive.

Reflection and Personal Application

We follow the life scripts written by others and established during childhood. These scripts are a set of instructions that tell us what to say, what we can and cannot do or what we should do. Like a movie, we are expected to follow the lines set down for us without deviation. While it lays the ground rules for how to interact with one another, they do not allow us to speak freely or have a genuine open discussion. Losses give us the opportunity to discard old scripts and rewrite new ones.

Throughout this journey, we have done the work necessary to make us stronger, self-reliant and caring. We have gone through the pain and healed emotional upheavals and exorcised old ghosts from the past. The stop button on repetitive, destructive and demeaning self-talk has been pushed and negative thinking has been replaced with positive thoughts and beliefs. We have developed optimism, flexibility and have given ourselves permission to be honest and real and we feel good about who we are.

A New Beginning: Setting Goals

Now it is time to actualize those new goals and aspirations. It is time to take those ideas and possibilities and put them into constructive goal statements with concrete plans of actions.

Any goal needs a definitive statement of what you want to accomplish and why. It requires a time frame of when you will start and designated completion. A plan of action is drawn up that defines the steps needed and what obstacles you may have to overcome along with a motivational program to keep you on track. The following helps explain these different parts.

Goal Statement

A goal statement simply defines in one or two sentences what you want to accomplish. Goals need to be personal and have value to you. They are not for someone else. When we have a long-held dream, we want to take that dream and make it into a goal that is both realistic and attainable. If it isn't specific and well defined, we may get discouraged and give up. Sometimes, larger goals need to be broken into small goals first.

The goal statement states exactly what you want to accomplish. If you want to become a teacher for example, your goal statement might say something like this: My goal is to complete an educational program and become a teacher.

Time Frame

Unless we establish a time frame with a definite starting and ending time, goals will simply remain wishes and dreams. We need both a written statement and a starting date to motivate us into action.

1. I will start ...
2. I hope to accomplish this by ...

Obstacles

Obstacles are anything that keep us from completing our goals or sabotaging our efforts. Identify as many of these as possible before you start. Make a list of ways you will overcome them. Here are some typical obstacles people face and ways to overcome them:

1. *Lack of faith and belief that I can accomplish it. I have failed in the past.*
   Overcome: I will make positive affirmations about my capability and read daily. I will remind myself of all the things I have accomplished.
2. *I don't have the funds to complete my goal.*
   Overcome: I will make a financial plan that includes a budget and securing a loan.

3. *Family support is important in completing any goals.*
   Overcome: Talk to them about why this goal is important to you. Listen to their concerns. Come to some agreement about how you can work together, share work details and support one another. Negotiate ways to meet their needs.

4. *What prior education and training do I have? Is it enough to begin my goal?*
   Overcome: Talk to college counselors; get information about various ways you can meet the requirements. There are many online courses available at all levels of education.

5. *What are the risks personally and emotionally?*
   Overcome: Sometimes the risks may seem overwhelming. Balance any risks with the rewards you will receive in completing your goal. Set up a plan for future pay off of expenses. Remind myself why this is important.

6. *What future obstacles will I face and how do I prepare for them?*
   Overcome: Think about possible setbacks and potential ways to handle these problems. "If this happens, I will do this..." What steps can you take now to prevent potential future problems?

7. Doubts can dampen enthusiasm and shake my belief that I can do this. Typical doubts include: *Am I good enough? Am I too old? What was I thinking? There is no way I can pull together the necessary resources.* Doubts focus on our limitations and need to be challenged immediately so we don't lose motivation and incentive. What we say to ourselves can become a self-fulfilling prophecy as we will act in accordance with self-talk.
   Overcome: In big, bold letters, write on a 3 x 5 card your goal and why it is important. Take other 3 x 5 cards and write affirmations that state your goal. Post them around the house where you will see them during the day. Stop and read them often. At the top of a card write, I can do this because.... then list all the things you have already accomplished.

Plan of Action

Create a step-by-step plan, like a to-do list, with the steps listed in the order needed to complete. This will eliminate forgetting any necessary steps. Cross them off as you complete each one.

Benefits

Unless you write down why your goal is important and the benefits that outweigh the risks, you will get discouraged and give up. Use your goal statement as an affirmation that you read each day as well.

Tracking

Goals take time to complete, and there will be times when we don't see any progress. But progress is measured by little steps. Each week evaluate what you have done and write down each accomplishment, no matter how minor or miniscule it may seem. Don't discredit or minimize the determination you used even when tired. You didn't give up. Reward yourself in some small way.

Be sensitive to the correctness of the goal itself. Is it still important to you? This is different than being discouraged. Sometimes we need to begin the process before we realize this isn't what you want after all. While we need to remain committed to our goals and not quit when we hit roadblocks or tough spots, it is also important to realize that completing a goal that is not right for you is a waste of time and energy.

Make a commitment and visualize your success

Make a formal commitment to yourself. Write it down, date it, and sign it. Visualize your success every day. Close your eyes and imagine what it will be like when you reach your goal. See yourself enjoying all the pleasant rewards of accomplishment.

Celebrate the completion of your goal with people who love and appreciate you and have supported you through this endeavor!

CHAPTER 24

A New Song and Dance

"I'm ready, God, so ready, ready from head to toe, ready to sing,
ready to raise a tune: Wake up, soul! Wake up, harp! Wake up
lute! Wake up, you sleepyhead sun! I'm thanking you, GOD,
out loud in the streets, singing your praises in town and
country. The deeper your love, the higher it goes;
every cloud is a flag to your faithfulness."

PSALM 57:7–10, *THE MESSAGE*

My heart is singing this morning. I am so ready to begin a new dance. I want to shed my clothes of mourning for good. I want to live!

As I enter a new phase of life as a single woman, I hear my internal voice say, "It's time to move forward. Take all the things you've learned on this journey and apply them in new goals and plans."

What have I learned? I've learned that I need the support of friends. I can survive most anything with the help of God and friends. I've learned to include God in all areas of my life and trust and believe that He is always there for me. I've learned that when I address pain head on, I can defuse its intensity and extract important messages that will enrich my life.

It takes time to go through the grieving process. It is important to grace ourselves time and patience while accepting the uncertainty of the future. There will be necessary moments of time spent in silence. For me, journaling every morning was a time of silence and communing with God, listening to his voice of comfort, strength, and courage. It is within silence where we can pour out our hearts without restraint. And when I did, I was able to let go and breathe in a new space.

A new dance of life! Exciting and full of promise and adventure! Where will tomorrow take me? I feel as though God is asking me to dance and that if I allow him to lead, he will teach me the steps of life that will hold peace, contentment, excitement, and happiness.

Walking with God can be risky, because I am not sure where it will lead me. I am required to trust. This is difficult for goal-oriented people like me. I am accustomed to taking control, deciding what I want to accomplish, removing obstacles, and making things happen. Now, I am including God in my planning.

I know that I can make plans and bring them about. But when I include God in the process, my plans have a better design full of stimulating, challenging, and enriching possibilities. It is both sobering and exciting to review options available to me for a new life.

Life! It's the ultimate dance. I can do it all alone, or I can ask God to be a partner. This exciting dance of life will require work, music, orchestration, discipline, and focus to learn the steps. But I am ready to go.

Reflection and Personal Application

How do we know when we are healed? We know we have finished grieving when we have fully accepted our losses. Some authors use phrases such as "weaving it into the fabric of our lives" or "reconciliation." I use phrases such as "coming to terms with" and "integrating" and "recovery."

When we have "come to terms" with our losses and accept what has happened emotionally as well as cognitively, they become integrated into our life stories. It does not mean that we won't have times of sorrow or anxiety or even depression. But it does mean that when pain no longer takes center stage, we will know we have recovered. We are able to talk about our loved ones with joy instead of sadness. A new plan will be designed to meet the demands of that unwanted chronic illness or that loss of limb. And we realize that divorce hasn't robbed us of who we are.

We gain confidence as we work on our goals and use new skills. As we master new proficiency, our losses are no longer a focal point. We rarely think about it; instead our focus is on fully developing who we are. As we accept a new normal, we have the assurance to step wholly and completely into that space.

Some things to consider as you experiment with this new phase in life:

1. Revisit your earlier list of past achievements. Then review the things you have learned on this journey. How have applying these new strengths and attributes made your life complete and whole again? Write a new description of who you are today.

2. Make a list of all the insights you have gained. These include new appreciation of traits and attributes you already had. Some things you have gained are fortitude, determination, strength, compassion, understanding, wisdom, and forgiveness. It took courage, perseverance and risk-taking; a willingness to make difficult choices, self-discipline, self-regulation, a new attitude, faith and belief in self and God. As you gain confidence you are able to trust your intuition and gut instincts. Add to this list.

Any new dance requires learning new steps. As you apply what you have learned, focus on what you can do, not what you can't. Take one step at a time; do one thing at a time. Rehearse it. Make it yours.

This is your dance; this is your new song! Together with the help of God, you are composing, arranging, and choreographing the steps you will need for your new dance of life. Winter is gone – Spring is here.

APPENDIX A

COMPLEX GRIEF EMOTIONS

L osses create emotional responses. We will experience many different and conflicting emotions while grieving. Circumstances can intensify and make it more difficult to work through some of them. The following three (anger, guilt, and shame) can create additional pain and conflict in our grieving and one may fuel the other. None of these emotions live in isolation but are intertwined with each other. A fourth, fear, can keep us immobilized from productively moving forward.

Anger

A loss resulting from carelessness, violence or some catastrophic disaster can create ongoing mental anguish directed to God or others. *Why me? What did I do to deserve this? We had waited so long for this child. I had always done what was right.* As we feel the sting of a harsh and indifferent reality, we find ourselves struggling over the unfairness of it all. Our belief system of natural expectation and justice has been violated.

If we feel we were the victims to such tragedies, anger can become a focal point in our grief. Without a way to direct that anger for moral reparation we often end up turning our anger into bitterness. As we rehearse over and over again our righteous indignation and anger, we construct a grievance story that continues to be played over and over again. The problem with such stories is we continue to inflict harm to ourselves. As Dr. Fred Luskin illustrates for us in his book, "Forgive for Good", grievances will eventually destroy us. Forgiveness allows us to let go of that pain. Otherwise we become its prisoner.

If we are the ones who made choices that harmed others in some way, whether perceived or in actuality, we can go from guilt to anger against ourselves that keep us locked in a negative cycle of self-blame. By inflicting self-recrimination and reproach over and over again, we receive some relief from our moral anger. Unable to forgive ourselves, we remain a prisoner to a cancer of the soul that slowly eats us up. *Why didn't I stay at the hospital with him instead of going home? Why did I say such things in anger? Why did I put her in a care facility? I should have seen the unhappiness and hopelessness that he was struggling with.* While we get short-term relief through self-incrimination, it is not a solution. Just as forgiveness releases us from pain inflicted on us by others, so forgiveness of self releases us from the on-going punishment we inflict on ourselves that will go nowhere. Only when we can become merciful to ourselves can we let go, accept absolution, and find peace.

When the faith we had in God now seems like a charade or pretense of what we believed, we may find ourselves angry and questioning God. *Why? I don't understand. If you really cared about us, how could you have allowed this to happen?* If we are unable to bring our anger to God in some sort of honest conversation, we will have difficulty finding resolution. When we pull away from what was a former source of comfort, anger can become deep-seated and turn into long-term bitterness and resentment.

Anger, like all emotions, has a purpose. It helps us survive and motivates us to take action and make important changes. Left unchecked, however, it becomes corrosive and will inflict additional pain and suffering on ourselves and others.

The above three examples of losses - senseless acts of others, a belief that we have made a bad choice and questioning our belief in God – can illustrate how easy it is to continue to fuel our anger and delay recovery.

Life is not only unfair; it is often cruel and heartless. As human beings, we struggle with injustice and trying to make sense of the nonsensical. There is a legitimate need to question incidents that go against our normal expectations of right and wrong. We have a right and need to get angry. But when we allow anger to become the directive of our life, it will not offer the relief and solutions you so desperately desire.

Here are three things to remember about anger:

- First, it is okay to be angry.
- Second, it is not okay to hurt yourself, someone else, or anyone's property.
- And third, we are responsible for what we do with our anger.

While venting or acting out might release some of anger's energy in the short term, it will not take away the source of it. If anger is your typical first response to unpleasant situations, you may have an anger problem. Professional counselors can help work through underlying causes.

Here are some constructive ways to deal with anger associated with grief:

1. Acknowledge your feelings of anger. Denying or pushing these feelings away only cause them to resurface later. Anger is a normal part of grieving.
2. Find a healthy way to release the immediate tension of anger. Pound a pillow or go to the gym and work out. Run. Walk. Move until the anger energy is released or reduced. Understand that while anger energy may have been reduced, the source of the anger will continue to fuel it unless addressed.
3. Talk about it. Find a supportive friend, pastor, or other nonjudgmental person who will listen as you share feelings and will give constructive feedback for clarification and validation. Oftentimes, talking things out is enough.

4. Write about it. Research indicates that as we write about it, we can lower its intensity and help us see a broader context. When the passion is reduced, thinking begins to moderate and we can work on ways to bring about resolution.

5. Challenge and change the thoughts and beliefs associated with anger. Reframe what has happened. Remove the sting. Coming to terms with senselessness, unfairness, and injustice can help us channel our energy in more positive ways. In the process, we will confront our own weaknesses and vulnerabilities and accept them as part of being human.

6. Accept. At some point, healing from grief and anger requires acceptance of what has happened, no matter how tragic or meaningless.

7. Take it to God. It is my personal belief that God is more capable of handling our anger than we are. He knows all about our anger and our susceptibility toward it. Consider the Psalms. The psalmist brings to God all his honest expressions of pain, anger, and questions, revealing a loving God who is compassionate and understanding of our foibles and frailties. If you are mad at God, tell him honestly and directly. "I am so angry at you for letting this happen." Talk to Him. Take your pain to Him. You may find deeper answers and a peace you so desire. When I come to God in honesty and humility, I am enriched beyond my expectations.

8. Make peace with what has happened. Find a good support group. A good grief and loss counselor or cognitive behavioral therapist can help you work through the tough parts. There may not be any answers that make sense no matter how much we want them to, but acceptance and forgiveness allows us to move on.

Guilt

Guilt is felt when our actions or lack of them are in opposition to what we believe we should do or is morally right. Feeling guilty is an indication that we may have done something wrong that requires making amends. Guilt is an emotion that gives us the opportunity to change directions or make amends. We learn in the process to think through options and make better decisions. When you have made amends, hanging onto guilt becomes a useless exercise.

Losses that create a sense of guilt for things we perceive as done or left undone can create a situation where there is no way to make amends. Along with internalized anger, we can use guilt to continue to beat ourselves up. We can become brutal in the self-blame game. Looking backward, we admonish ourselves, "If only I had done this or that" or "If only I had been more available."

While asking questions and searching for appropriate answers are important, it serves no purpose to continue in an ongoing cycle of guilt, shame, or remorse. Remaining in a state of blame only adds another intense layer of pain to our grief. Working through guilt is working through the many "what if's" and "if only's" and putting them to rest.

Here are some of the typical questions that initiate and perpetuate guilt:

- What if I had spent more time listening and being involved? Would I have seen the warning signs of depression and despair and been able to stop the suicide?
- What if I hadn't put my spouse in a nursing home where she felt rejected, abandoned, and unhappy? Would her final days have been better?
- What if I hadn't said such hurtful things just before he left for work?
- What if my friend had lived and I had died instead?
- If only I had insisted he go to the doctor sooner; the cancer might have been treatable.
- If only I hadn't gone out with friends, I would have been able to call 911.

LEARNING TO LIVE AGAIN IN A NEW WORLD

- If only I hadn't been so abrasive, maybe he would not have left home angry and the accident wouldn't have happened.

Along with the "what if's" and "if only's" come questions of why, such as:

- Why did God allow this? It is so unfair and makes no sense.
- Why did he have to die at this time when we had our whole life ahead of us?
- Why did she die in the crash while I lived?
- Why didn't I use better judgment or make better decisions?

These questions and many others leave us feeling angry, guilty, frustrated, and helpless. Expanding and reframing what happened help give us a different perspective.

- Could I really have done anything different?
- What information do I have today that I didn't have back then?
- Am I taking responsibility for other people's actions?
- Is my guilt a way to ease some of the pain of the loss itself?
- Is guilt keeping me from grieving my loss, letting go, and moving forward?

Responsible and moral individuals struggle with wrongs, perceived or otherwise, they may have perpetuated or initiated. Once again, guilt can help us think more carefully, but we need to forgive ourselves and move forward.

Shame

Guilt and shame go hand in hand. Shame is an intense emotion of regret we feel when we recognize we have done something wrong. Guilt, along with shame, helps us say we are sorry and ask for forgiveness. It allows us to say we regret what we have done. It is important to acknowledge and respond appropriately to both.

But when faced with losses that occur outside the normal expectations we hold and put enormous pressure and uncertainty on us, we may be plagued with a guilt and consequent shame afterwards that may be misplaced, prolonged, or even inappropriate to the situation. Once again, 20-20 hindsight gives us additional information to respond differently. John Bradshaw has worked a lifetime to help us understand the elements of shame and I highly recommend reading the two books I have referenced if you are dealing with ongoing shame.

When guilt disproportionate to any actions we may have taken continues to dominate our thinking, it becomes toxic. If we have overreacted to our sense of responsibility for actions taken or not taken, our shame for perceived transgressions may be out of proportion to what occurred. By remaining in a state of on-going guilt and shame, it will eventually erode our sense of self as caring, compassionate and honorable individuals. Guilt and shame that exceeds our ability to have been responsible will eventually corrode our abilities to live productive and fruitful lives.

Coming to terms with any loss means we come to terms with ourselves as human beings. If guilt is appropriate to the event, such as driving drunk and hurting somebody, then we can use that guilt as a precursor to turning our lives around. When possible, say you're sorry to people you have offended and then take actions to make amends when possible.

Hanging onto feelings of guilt and shame, nursing them in order to do penance, doesn't change anything; instead, it keeps us from productive living. Forgiveness enables us to take positive action instead of remaining in an unchangeable past.

Go ahead and ask the questions that are troubling you, but then be realistic as you challenge your responses. It is important to remember that we make the best decisions we can in any moment in time based on who we are and the information we have. Anyone can look backward and see things we didn't see in the moment.

Here are a couple of things you can do that can help alleviate the strong emotions associated with guilt and shame.

1. Write a letter to the person who died. Tell him/her all the things you wish you could have done, what you wanted to have happen, and how you feel. Tell that person you love him/her and that you are letting go of all the "what if's and if only's" and you are releasing and absolving any remaining guilt.
2. Write a letter to yourself. Dear ... (Put in your name). Tell yourself that you have done your best and that you are extending grace and forgiveness to yourself.

Fear

Change of any kind creates anxiety. What was familiar is no more. We haven't been in this situation before and do not know what to expect. Losses can have severe and far-reaching consequences to our life that was unexpected and many times unwarranted. Such events create anxiety and fear.

Like anger, fear is an emotion of survival. It prepares us to either fight or flee from any situation that might be a source of danger. Losses put us in life changes that can create a similar feeling about our survival for the future. If you lost a spouse, went through an ugly divorce or no longer have the health to earn an income, it is a frightening and daunting feeling. If your loss was associated with bad planning and unexpected financial turn of events, we may feel shock and then anxiety and fear. What do I do now? Ongoing fear with no resolution can become aggravated and make it very difficult to make the decisions needed.

The loss I encountered put me in such a financial bind. Because of the suddenness and untimely death of my husband, the pension we depended on stopped. We had just built our dream home and had a small home mortgage. I was required to sell my home. My daughter developed breast cancer less than a year after his death and I had a degenerating hip, which required surgery. These were not things we could have anticipated ahead of time, but which created a number of challenges for me along with my grief. I had to examine all the options available and then choose the best one. Going through the process was difficult but strengthening and rewarding.

A divorce can create a lot of anxiety as well. Can I work with a spouse who abandoned me with issues of child custody, visitations, etc.? Will I have enough money to remain in my home and raise the children? Who can I depend on? Will I ever be able to trust again?

We feel vulnerable when life hands us a truck full of troubles at one time and we become afraid. It is important that we respond to what fear is telling us, especially if there is imminent physical danger of some kind. If it is financial danger, we need to put emergency measures in place as soon as possible. Facing our fears help us to look for solutions and put them in place.

But our fears can be embellished and out of proportion to any real danger. Without a visible target for our fear, we need to ask: "Why am I afraid? Why am I panicked or worried?" Dangers real or imaginary need to be faced and specially defined. If we just have a fear of the unknown and the uncertainty associated with that, exploring our reasons to be afraid can be freeing. There are always solutions of some kind.

As you address feelings of ongoing, undefined fear, ask yourself what is motivating those feelings of anxiety and fear. Would additional information regarding a life altering decision help reduce some of that fear? Seek out people who can give you information or who can mentor you. Are you feeling inadequate and don't trust yourself? If so, work on exercises that promote your innate ability to find the solutions that are right for you. Everyone needs to ask for help.

Fear is a good thing. It teaches us to be cautious and not take life for granted. It can teach us to initiate preventive measures in how we live. In grief, we may experience an inappropriate or inflated ongoing fear that can isolate us. It is important to identify what is creating those fears and causing the most anxiety so we can address them specifically. The more you can be honest with yourself, the more you will be able to trust your judgment and ability to make sound decisions. This can be a turning point in your life where you discover your need for God and for others. As we experience genuine humility, we can both respect and learn from our fears.

Some things to consider:

- Fear is a survival mechanism. It protects and warns us of potential danger.
- Fear tells us to stop and be cautious—it is not to be ignored.
- Fear supplies the adrenalin to act.
- Fear tells us to prepare.
- Fear reveals our insecurities.
- Fear tells us we are not sufficient unto ourselves.
- Fear can drive us to God (see Psalm 91, "God, you're my refuge").
- Fear will challenge us.
- Fear can motivate us.
- Fear can help us grow.

All emotions give us valuable information that we need to live, survive, and thrive. They are all necessary and beneficial and have a purpose. If we will allow them to help direct and monitor our behaviors and challenge outdated and inappropriate beliefs, we will gain appreciation for ourselves and our world.

APPENDIX B

SUPPORT SYSTEMS

E ach person will mourn from their own unique perspective, their personality style, and what that loss meant to them personally. Some people are comfortable talking about their feelings while others find it awkward and would rather withdraw from social interactions and reflect in silence. It is often difficult for spouses to share or talk about what they are experiencing but find it easier to talk with friends.

Whether you withdraw or find solace in disclosure, we all need support. While one person may find great comfort in laughter and sharing stories about the person they lost, another may find any expression of pleasure too painful. Some people may fear laughter might be construed as their loss not having the value it did. Understanding how your friend, spouse, or family member mourns will be helpful in giving the support that is needed.

There are no determined rules about mourning, although we may have grown up with certain cultural rituals. When helping those who are grieving, avoid imposing your personal beliefs about perceived do's and don'ts onto another, unless self-destructive behaviors are present. If we put expectations or restrictions on how a mourner ought to act, or when they should be through grieving, we can make their recovery more difficult and drive their sorrow underground. Subtle suggestions, which imply that if you only had more faith or more trust in God than you would be in less pain, only compounds the emotional and mental suffering.

When listening and comforting someone, we often share our own experiences with loss. While this may let the mourner know they are not alone in their tragedy and that we understand what they are going through, it could be a deterrent if the emphasis is switched from their story to our own. While tragedies and situations may be similar, each is unique within the context of personal definition. The depth of pain and complexities involved will be different for each person.

Support for Those We Love and Care About

Friends offer a unique support system for the mourner. As a friend, we can often anticipate and offer assistance while being sensitive to their needs without becoming intrusive. We can't take away the pain, but we can walk beside them while they go through it.

In the early months of my grief, my friends were an integral part of my healing. They helped me reenter the social world I had shared with them before the death of my husband. Their actions said to me, "You are still one of us, you are our friend, and we weep with you." This is important because in many situations your loss will affect the social network you had.

Over time, some friendships will remain strong while others diminish. But that is the normal course of relationships and not exclusive to the drastic change that has taken place in your life. When I was grieving, my friends were instrumental in helping me when the pain was most intense. Such support is immeasurable and worth more than any words or monetary value one might place upon it. Friends help normalize the process as we work through the many layers.

Here are some ways to support a friend who is grieving:

1. Be accessible. Don't wait for the grieving person to call you. When they do, try to respond as quickly as possible. Emotional pain can make a person feel vulnerable, making it difficult to

ask for help. They may not want to be a burden on others. Many times, individuals who are grieving do not know what they want beyond the basics of life such as food, etc. Stay in touch and check in periodically to see how they are doing.

2. Be specific about your assistance. "May I come and help you on Saturday? I'm going to the store and would love to have your company. May I pick you up at ...? I set an extra place at the table, and we want you to come and join us for dinner." Or perhaps just invite them to go for a walk.

3. Be empathetic. Empathy is not sympathy or pity. Empathy is putting yourself in the other's shoes and walking with them as they move through a troubling time. Compassion can be expressed with a brief embrace, a hug, or touch on the shoulder, a squeeze of the hand, or a willingness to just be there and listen. Treat them as a normal person. Pity destroys self-respect and adds to the pain.

4. Honor their space. Conflicting and intense emotions can make it difficult to talk about feelings, as it is often difficult to put into words. They may feel defenseless and exposed and want to withdraw. Respect that vulnerability as you keep in touch. Not everyone wants to talk and not everyone wants to be drawn out. Let them know you care. You can be sensitive and available without putting pressure on them to talk. Retreat, however, can become isolation. Invite them to join you in projects you have enjoyed and shared in the past or ask them to join you in a new class or group. Be willing to expand what you do to include them when possible.

5. Validate feelings. Feelings will vary from situation to situation and individual to individual. Some people might feel intense anger—at God, the world, themselves, life—while others simply feel an overwhelming sense of sadness. *Validate* means to confirm, endorse, or authenticate what they are experiencing. Be sensitive to the space they are in. Don't presume to know

the depth of their grief. Don't be afraid of tears. It is part of the grieving and healing process.

6. Be a good listener. Listening requires being present in the moment. A good listener will acknowledge the thoughts and feelings of another by giving feedback without judgment of what is being said and observed. Focus on the person and not the responses you want to make. Example: "It must be difficult to put into words what you are feeling right now. I can see you are hurting." Open the door to conversation but let the mourner lead. Accept silence as well as conversation.

7. Temper any counsel. It is difficult to listen without offering advice. But it is important to moderate any advice or solutions we want to offer. Your advice may not be right for them. Avoid intellectualizing.

8. Be a trusted friend. Whatever is said to you in confidence is not to be shared or judged. Again, people who grieve can feel very vulnerable. They are not only experiencing intense and often conflicting and confusing emotions, but also conflicting thoughts and memories. If the mourner has thoughts of suicide, however, strongly encourage them to seek professional help and keep in close contact with them.

9. Help normalize life. Use the name of the person who died. Avoiding discussion about death can minimize the importance of that person to the griever. You don't have to probe for details. Give them a safe place to share and offer information if they want it. Listen with understanding.

Support will have more value when we have confronted our own beliefs about loss, death, and dying. Being embarrassed with the expression of our emotions, personal pain, and helplessness can make it uncomfortable for others around you. When we face and accept our own mortality and emotional response to that, it will be easier to reach out with compassion and understanding.

When Listening Isn't Enough

Each is required to work through the problems of life and find solutions that are right for us. When asked for advice or help from another, clarify the problem by asking questions. When offering recommendations or counsel, remember we are helping find solutions that are appropriate for others, not ourselves.

There is a difference between listening empathetically and enabling. The first helps move the griever through their pain to resolution. The second enables them to remain stuck. When someone continues to repeat the same behaviors over and over with no visible evidence of moving forward, listening may not be enough. It is appropriate to suggest they seek the help of a good grief counselor.

Support alone may not offer the resolutions wanted or needed. But it does affirm the griever's journey and offers that encouragement to "hang in there." It suggests that each of us has that internal strength deep within us to overcome any adversity.

At some point, those who are supporting others will be required to set boundaries for themselves. If you are listening to the continuous lament of someone who is not working through their grief, it might be helpful to respond like this: "I know you are hurting, and I want to support you, but I can't help you through this pain. Please get some assistance from a pastor, counselor, or support group."

Or you may need to be more firm: "I want to continue to be friends, but your comments continue to bring my spirits down. I know you are hurting, and I want to help you enjoy life again. Let's talk about ways to make life good again."

Comments and Statements to Avoid

It is often difficult to know what to say to someone who is grieving. We feel their intense ache and want to help relieve some of that suffering. What we say does make a difference.

We may be tempted to repeat clichés we have heard in the past as we struggle to find those comforting words. The things we say do have the power to diminish or minimize what the mourner is experiencing. Caring and compassion are different than feeling sorry for someone. The words we use can reflect this.

The following are suggested statements offered by professionals and researchers and taken from a multitude of sources and publications in the field of grief and loss that we avoid saying to people in our attempts to comfort them:

- *I know it will be hard, but time will heal.*
- *He lived a long life.*
- *It was God's will.*
- *I know exactly how you feel.*
- *You are still young; you can have another baby.*
- *Be thankful you have other children.*
- *All things must pass.*
- *You will find somebody else again.*
- *Be grateful you had him/her so long.*
- *You will feel better in a few weeks.*
- *She/he isn't hurting anymore.*
- *It must have been his/her time.*

These and other time-worn or spiritual statements can be confusing, conflicting, insensitive, untrue, and in general unhelpful. Substitute them for statements such as

- *It's hard to understand why these things happen.*
- *Your pain seems overwhelming.*
- *This must be very painful and hard for you.*
- *I can't imagine what you are feeling or experiencing.*
- *I am sorry for your loss.*

Avoid explaining what has happened in the hope of relieving pain such as:

- *There must be a purpose.*
- *He lived a long life.*
- *It's God's will.*
- *He is out of pain now.*

Wounded people need

- Love and acceptance, not judgment
- A hand up, not a handout
- Compassion, not pity
- Time to heal, to be alone, and to be with others
- Someone to listen to them
- Understanding and validation

EPILOGUE

It may seem that your journey never ends. And in many ways, it is ongoing as you explore new options and test new avenues to bring joy, love and contentment back into your life. It is easy to get discouraged. If you think of this as a new journey that is connected with the one you are leaving behind, you allow for new unexpected surprises of hope and happiness to reveal themselves.

Working through the chapters of this book, you dealt with the twists and turns of conflicting emotions and confronted questions that had no easy or satisfactory answers.

As you let go of old assumptions and expectations you began reassembling the pieces of your life and moved into creating a new meaningful beginning. You redefined who you were and stepped out in confidence.

There will be times when you feel you are back in the grieving mode. But as you continue to explore, examine and reassemble the pieces of your life, you will be able to forge them into a new satisfying reality. You will not only find solace and comfort in revisiting your memories but will be able to celebrate the life of your loved one. They will always be with you.

Losses give us pause to consider more than just the ordinary; it allows us to consider and examine what is meaningful in life and then find new ways to establish that again. It is a time of renewal. And you are in the driver's seat.

Additional Resources

Your local Hospice is a wonderful organization that offers support and help to people as they go through this journey. Most hospitals offer support groups that you can join. There are other more specific groups such as The Compassionate Friends, an international support group for grieving parents, especially those who lost a child to crime or trauma who may have a local chapter in your vicinity. Cornerstone of Hope is another large organization which offers support, education, counseling and art therapy for children, teens and adults who are grieving. Check with your local chamber of commerce, hospital or church for chapters and support groups in your location. Loss is a wounding that needs the support, care, and understanding from those who can relate to it, have worked through it, and can help you go through it.

Study Guide
Use with Groups

Chapter 1 – This Can't be Happening

During those early days and weeks, emotions and thoughts go from shock to this can't be happening. Writing is very helpful. Start a journal and record what you are experiencing. What are some ways you can offer yourself compassion and comfort?

Chapter 2 – Alice's Surreal World.

You may have had to go back to work with little time off. List some ways you can make time to grieve, whether alone or with others.

Chapter 3 – A Psalm of Tears

Grieving takes you into times of extreme sorrow and other times when things seem normal. What can help as you go through the ups and downs of this time? Look at the list of suggestions in your book and try some. Start a gratitude journal and write down something every day that you are grateful for no matter how small. How can you find ways to bring laughter into your day?

Chapter 4 – On Eagle's Wings – Let go and Soar

Grief is hard work. It can be overwhelming and exhausting. Practicing mindfulness and relaxation techniques are both restful and healing. Use the relaxation script at the end of this study guide to help you relax individually or use in a group setting.

Chapter 5 – That Still Small Voice

Losses are like an onion with layers to be unwrapped. What unexpected layers are you discovering with your loss? Pain can isolate us. How do you include others in your life? What is most difficult when you are with others?

Chapter 6 – Prayer

Prayer is acting as if God were there with you all the time. Are you able to communicate with God and develop a more personal relationship? If not, what holds you back?

Chapter 7 – And God said Rest

Resting is stopping the frantic "doing" and just "be", reflecting and staying focused in the moment. Using the Relaxation Exercise in Chapter 4, add different visualizations. Which ones bring you the most comfort? What are you discovering about yourself through these exercises?

Chapter 8 – Battles (depression)

Depression often sets in while trying to let go of what was. Schedules and routines can offset feelings of depression. Chaotic environments feed anxiety, while routines help establish normalcy and stability. If you struggle with drugs, alcohol or food, keep a daily log to reveal a pattern of when the most difficult time of day is for you. What pleasant things can you reward yourself with to replace the urge to self-medicate?

Chapter 9 – Blessed are the Poor in Spirit

Psychological and emotional pain has a purpose. It protects and helps us survive by telling us something is not right; we need to pay attention, make corrections, change directions, slow down or take a time out. Pain often includes feelings of guilt, anger, rejection, bitterness, deep sorrow as well as depression. What are you learning about yourself, your world and how God is working through your sorrow to help you become more resilient, compassionate and strong? Congratulate yourself for all your hard work and progress.

Chapter 10 – Let God Lead

Emotions give us information. What intense emotions such as anger, guilt or shame are you struggling with? Keep a record for a week to discover when these are triggered, and the thoughts associated with them. Are you able to challenge those negative thoughts and replace them with constructive ones? Here is one example, "I am so angry that the car accident took the life of my loved one." Challenge, reframe and replace with, "I am angry, but it is time to let go and do something constructive to help and support myself and others." Review the list in Appendix A. Do you recognize yourself in any of them?

Chapter 11 – Acceptance

Acceptance is a difficult concept. What thoughts and feelings are making it difficult to accept and let go? What part of your loss do you continue to struggle with and what needs to happen to release yourself? Letting go is a conscious choice. When we can let go, we can build a bridge to a new beginning.

Chapter 12 - The Struggle to Believe

What major decision are you facing right now? Example: a move, a new career, financial concerns, etc.? Make a list of each problem, potential solutions, risks and benefits. Decisions made to escape uncomfortable feelings will often be bad decisions. What emotions are you struggling with as you make new important decisions?

Chapter 13 – A Time to Laugh and a Time to Cry

The season of loss is also a season of discovery. As we let go of struggles and questions that have no logical answers, we can focus on the here and now. Start a new journal entitled, A New Beginning. Write down all the new things you are discovering about yourself? Example: resiliency, flexibility, tolerance, faith, courage, trust, hope, etc. Be honest and nonjudgmental.

Chapter 14 – Entwining Roots

In a Remembrance Book add pieces of life shared before your loss, such as old letters, birth certificates, or anything that "captures" the spirit of your loved one. Include your writing. Expressions of love have formed some incredible pieces of literature written by individuals who were not writers but simply expressing the love they shared through grief. In the act of writing, the spirit creates the words we need. Create a wall hanging or collage or a memory quilt. Following the example and instructions in this chapter, write a letter to your loved one.

Chapter 15 – Smoke and Mirrors

As we process our loss, we are making a transition from what was to what is now. Reflect on the dreams you had in the past. Is this something you want to revisit? What obstacles need to be overcome to complete your goal? Write a letter to yourself following the instructions in this chapter. Do you find yourself using critical self-talk? How can you replace these statements?

Chapter 16 – Path? What Path?

Endings can be scary. To walk a new path requires expanding your horizon and trying new things. Are there things in your past that keep you stuck? What fears keep interfering? What old beliefs, lifestyles, life scripts, assumptions, expectations, etc. are keeping you from exploring new options? Give yourself permission to explore who you want to become.

Chapter 17 – Seagulls on the Wind

Use the script to help yourself or the group you are leading relax and then follow with this visualization. Then, discuss the potentials for them as they apply this to their lives.

See yourself walking along the beach. Look around and see items that the sea tossed on the shore. Are there some items that capture your attention? Imagine picking up these pieces, some broken or worn smooth by pounding waves, and taking them home. As you visualize how to display them, see yourself creating an attractive sculpture, arrangement, wall hanging or picture from them. Then, step back and enjoy what you have created.

Imagine that this new creation is you. You are that magnificent treasure. What was tenderly reworked, sculpted or re-arranged with great care and love? What did you add to enhance this work of art? Stand back and see yourself as this newly fashioned work of art, woven into a beautiful new sculpture or a rich tapestry of old and new. Hang this beautiful new portrait of "you" filled with hope, wisdom and high regard, on the wall of your mind. Then open your eyes and return to the present moment.

Chapter 18 – In the Storm of Life

Losses often come in bunches – we have barely recovered when we are struck again. Old losses from our past are often triggered. What losses from your past have you remembered? Using the information in your book, can you challenge the validity of these old messages? What affirmations can you create to draw you towards a more productive and affirming future?

Chapter 19 – Therapy of Writing

Writing or journaling helps to clarify and heal. What insights have you gained through this journey that will help you moving forward? What are some of the destructive comments your internal critic has made? Using the examples given, challenge your internal critic and replace with affirming statements.

Chapter 20 – My Special Place

Reflecting on past accomplishments helps us conquer adversity today. It reminds us we not only survived but thrived. What are some of your past accomplishments and how were you able to overcome adversity to achieve them? Do you recognize your strengths? How does this encourage you?

Chapter 21 – Surrounded by Blessings

Losses give us an opportunity to appreciate more of our life. It takes life as usual and reveals the extraordinary. It is a place of awareness and shifting from pain to appreciation and excitement for the future. Do you give yourself permission to acknowledge and celebrate the things you are grateful for?

Chapter 22 – On top of the Mountain

When we have traveled those tough paths up a mountain we are rewarded at the top with an expansive view of possibilities. Loss may give us short pause in the scheme of things; but it allows us to consider and examine what a meaningful life means. How can you take charge of your life? What options for your future have you considered?

Chapter 23 – A Fresh Start

Revisit your earlier list of past achievements. Give yourself credit for all your efforts as well as any achievements. Make a list of all the traits and attributes that were needed to achieve those goals. What new attributes have you acquired since your loss, or appreciation for life? Following the steps in this chapter, construct a simple goal with a definitive plan of action.

Chapter 24 – A New Song and Dance

You have acquired a new appreciation of yourself, your journey and your future. Some closing thoughts: review everything you have learned. Make a list of all the things you have learned and gained on this journey. How will you apply them in the future? How will you continue to encourage and motivate yourself? Write a mission statement of the values you want to live by.

Relaxation script for individuals and group setting

If you are by yourself, find a quiet spot where you will not be disturbed and sit comfortably in a chair with hands in your lap and feet on the floor. If you have small children, be sure they are attended to. This exercise takes only about ten to fifteen minutes. Start small and expand as you become comfortable with relaxing.

1. Close your eyes and start breathing deeply and evenly. Avoid shallow chest breathing. Instead, feel your diaphragm move in and out with each breath, as you breathe in through the nose and exhale slowly through the mouth. After you practice this a few times, you will notice your heart rate slowing to a steady and even rhythm and tension being released from your muscles. Just focusing on your breathing, the diaphragm rising and falling and how your body feels in response is relaxing.

2. As you allow your mind to relax, thoughts about what you should or ought to be doing try to capture your attention. Unless you are reminded of something urgent, such as the care and safety of your children, simply redirect your attention to your breathing. Do not resist or try to force thoughts away. This only increases tension. Instead, continue to focus on your steady breathing allowing thoughts to float away. Intruding thoughts can be very persistent and demanding. With practice, however, it becomes easier and easier to remain focused in the here and now.

3. As you relax, focus on the different parts of your body, breathe into that spot and let go of the tension. With practice you will feel the muscles relax whenever you breathe deeply and tell yourself to let go.

4. When your breathing and relaxation practice has deepened, you can expand your relaxation with visualization. Our brain responds to pictures and symbols. Visualization is simply allowing your mind to produce positive mental imagery and pleasing pictures, either from old experiences or creating new ones. These can produce feelings of safety, deep relaxation, and peace and enhance healing. When our minds focus on hurtful and painful images, the opposite is true: we experience tension, anxiety, and helplessness.

   Along with the positive mental pictures and images our brain produces, we are able to experience an entire range of sensory effects when deeply relaxed: the weightlessness of a soaring eagle or the warmth of a sandy beach. We can recall the smells of the ocean or pine forest or the sweet scent of flowers without any allergic reaction. Think back to times when you experienced peace and deep contentment; focus on these memories when you are relaxed.

   Create specific visualizations that have importance to you. Mediate on your favorite Scripture verses of promise and comfort or encouraging words of others. Fashion images in your mind that focus on healing, such as visualizing lying in a warm, soothing pool of water. As you relax, feel the aches and pains drain away.

5. When you have finished your relaxation and visualization exercise, count from three to one in your mind and open your eyes. Stretch your muscles and remain sitting for a few minutes before getting up for circulation to energize you again.

Marlene Anderson, M.A.

Selected Readings
and References

Over the course of my own personal healing and recovery, I have read many books on grief and loss and completed over fifty professional continuing education hours on the topic. While writing this book, I drew from my own experiences and professional training as a licensed therapist, along with many clinical and therapy books. Although there were many resources (too many to include here), the list below is some of the references I have specifically drawn from. All of them have added in some way to understanding the process of grief and ways we can work with it.

Amen, Daniel G., M.D., *Change Your Brain, Change your Body*, 3 Rivers Press, N.Y.2010

American Art Therapy Association; www.arttherapy.org; attended *Art Therapy for Grief and Loss*, Marylhurst University, Margaret Hartsook, MA, BFA, ATR, 2009

Beck, Judith S. *Cognitive Behavior Therapy, Second Edition: Basics and Beyond*. Guilford Press, 2011

Bonnano, George A. *The Other Side of Sadness: What the New Science of Bereavement Tells Us about Life After Loss*. Basic Books, 2010.

Bradshaw, John, *Healing the Shame that Binds You*. Deerfield Beach, Florida, Health Communications, Inc. 1933

Bradshaw, John. *Reclaiming Virtue.* NY, Bantam Dell, A Division of Random House, 2009

Bridges, William. *Transitions: Making Sense of Life's Changes.* Da Capo Press, 2004.

Cook, Alicia Skinner and Dworkin, Daniel S. *Helping the Bereaved: Therapeutic Interventions for Children, Adolescents, and Adults.* Basic Books, 1992

Cameron, Julia with Bryan, Mark. *The Artist's Way: A Spiritual Path to Higher Creativity. Journaling Strategies.* New York, Putnam Book, 2002

De Becker, Gavin, *The Gift of Fear,* Dell Publishing, 1007

De Foore, Bill, Ph.D., *Anger, Deal with it, heal with it, Stop it from Killing You,* Health Communications, Inc., Deerfield Beach, Florida, 1991

Ellis, Albert, Ph.D., *Anger: How to Live with and Without it,* Carol Publishing Group, 1990

James, John W & Friedman, Russell Friedman. *Grief Recovery Handbook.* Harper Perennial, 2009

Jantz, Gregory, L. PhD, and Ann MacMurray, *Moving Beyond Depression,* Waterbrook Press, 2003

Leech, Peter, MSW, LCSW & Singer, Zeva, MA, MFCC. *Acknowledgment: Opening to the Grief of Unacceptable Loss.* Wintercreek Publications, 1990

Loewinsohn, Ruth Jean, *Survival Handbook for Widows and for Relatives and Friends Who Want to Understand.* AARP, 1984

Luskin, Dr. Fred. *Forgive for Good.* New York, New York, Harper Collins, 2002

Klein, Allen. *The Healing Power of Humor,* Jeremy Tarcher/Putnam, Inc, NY. 1989

Konigsberg, Ruth Davis, *The Truth about Grief,* Simon & Schuster, Ny. Ny 2011

Kosminsky, Phyllis, PhD. *Getting Back to Life When Grief Won't Heal,* McGraw Hill, 2007

McKay, Matthew Ph.D., Rogers, Peter D., Ph.D., McKay, Judith, R.N., edited by Kirk Johnson. *When Anger Hurts,* New Harbinger Publications, Inc., 1989

O'Connor, Nancy Ph.D. *Letting Go with Love: The Grieving Process,* La Mariposa Press, 2007

Oregon Counseling Association, 1992 Fall Conference, *Moving Through Grief and Loss, Understanding the Many Losses we all face*

Rando, Therese A. *Grief, Dying, and Death: Clinical Interventions,* Research Press, 1984

Richman, Linda. *I'd Rather Laugh: How to Be Happy Even When Life Has Other Plans for You* Warner Books, 2001

Smith, Harold Ivan, *When You Don't Know What to Say, how to help your grieving friends,* Beacon Hill Press of Kansas City, Kansas City, Missouri 2002

Tavris, Carol. *Anger, The Misunderstood Emotion,* Touchstone Press, 1989

Wolfelt, Alan D., Ph.D. *Healing a Spouse's Grieving Heart 100 Practical Ideas After Your Husband or Wife Dies,* Healing Your Grieving Heart Series, Companion Press 2003

Wolfelt, Alan, Ph.D. *The PTSD Solution,* Companion Press, 2015

Worthington, Jr., edited by. *Dimension of Forgiveness, Psychological Research & Theological Perspectives,* Templeton Foundation Press, 1998

Yancy, Philip, *Where is God when it Hurts,* Zondervan, 1990

BIOGRAPHY

Marlene Anderson is a licensed mental health counselor, author, speaker and retreat/workshop leader. She has worked in clinical, educational, business and church settings, as a college teacher and facilitator of psycho-educational classes. She has developed and delivered course material on diverse subjects including parenting, stress management, pain management, grief and loss and communication.

Marlene is the author of *"A Love so Great, A Grief so Deep"*, and contributing author to *"It's A God Thing"* and *"Heaven Touching Earth"*, available on Amazon.com. Her latest relaxation CD is available on her website along with her book, *"Use Stress to Meet Your Goals"*. You can follow her weekly blogs and podcasts on her website, www.focuswithmarlene.com. Marlene can be contacted through her e-mail info@focuswithmarlene.com.

CPSIA information can be obtained
at www.ICGtesting.com
Printed in the USA
LVHW032048210120
644359LV00006B/53

9 781400 329366